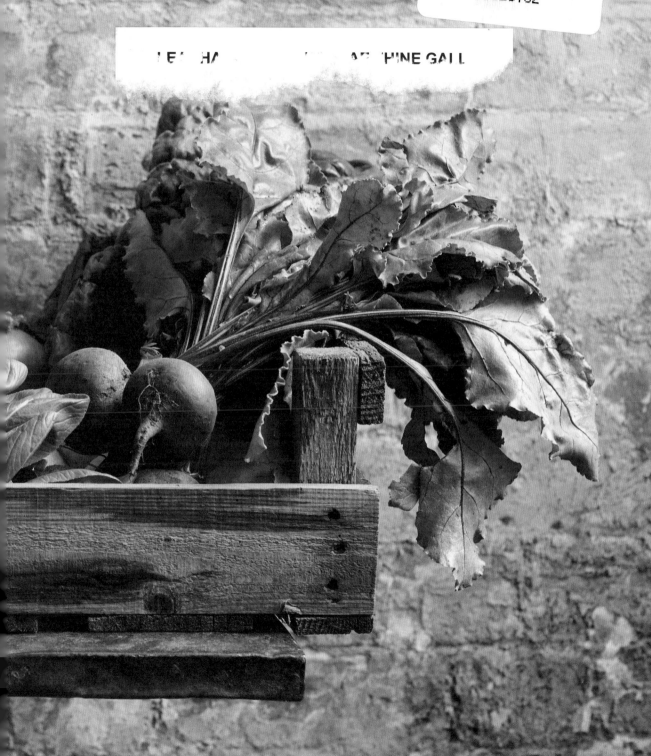

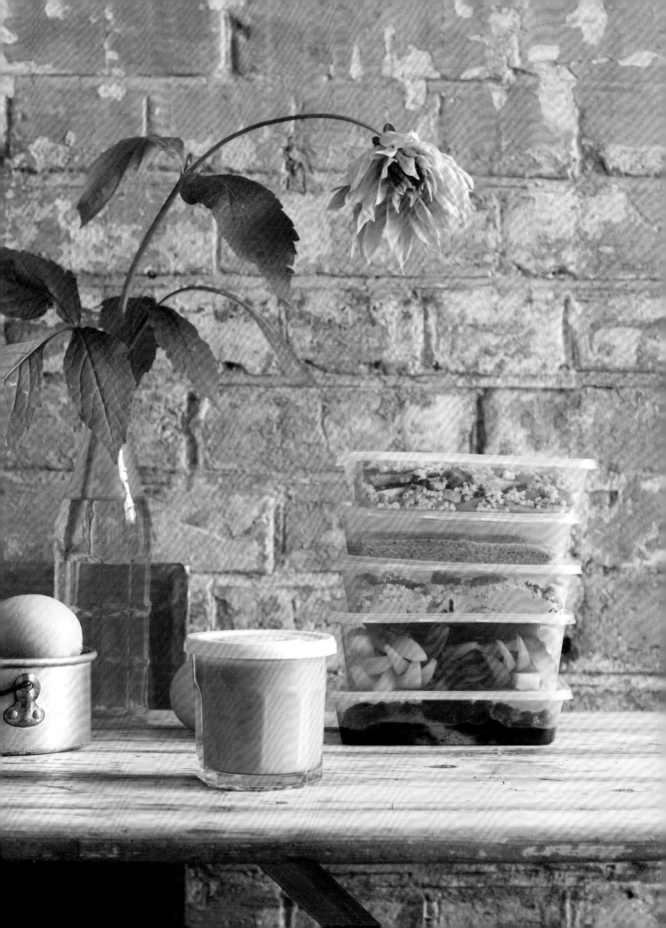

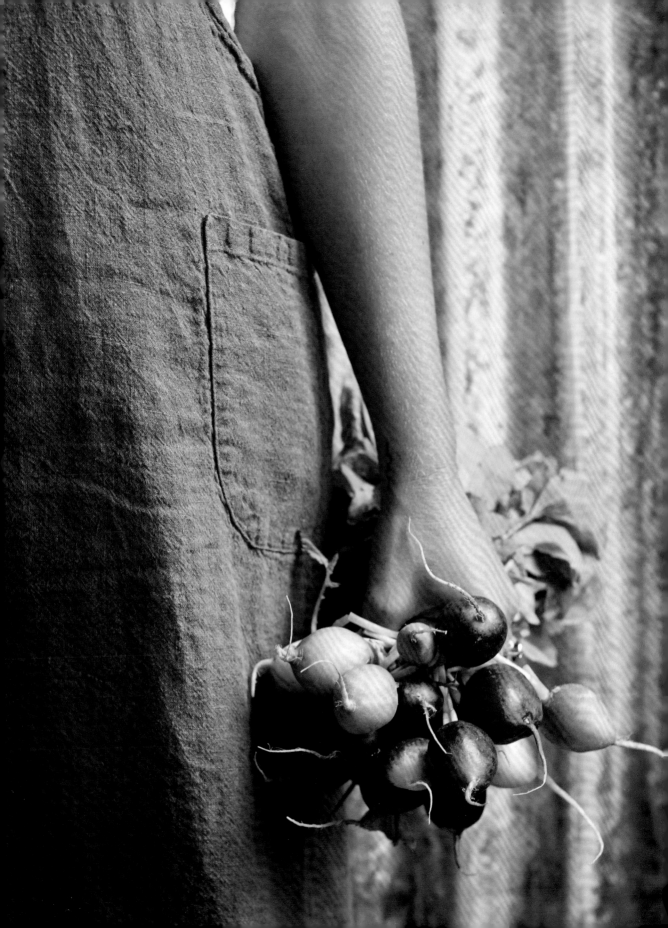

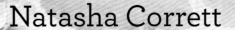

Natasha Corrett

HONESTLY HEALTHY

in a hurry

The busy food-lover's cookbook

HODDER &
STOUGHTON

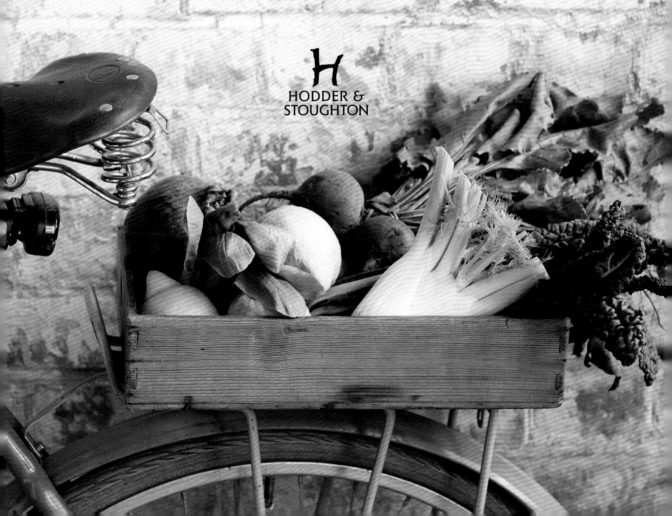

To Simon, my husband,
your love inspires me to be the
best person I can. Thank you
for always being hungry so I had
to learn to cook healthily
in a hurry!

contents

introduction

'By failing to prepare, you are preparing to fail.'
BENJAMIN FRANKLIN

**Starting the day in a hurry and running out of your home
without eating breakfast is one of the worst things you can do to your
health. It sets you off on a bad foot for the rest of your day, causing
unhealthy habits to arise. However, if you have delicious, nutritious food
ready prepared in your fridge, you can grab something on the
way out of the door and set yourself up for the day.**

Being in a hurry can be the result of poor time management, which I most definitely have. Not planning my time properly and thinking I can squeeze in one more meeting or project, ends up meaning I eat into 'my' time. Being in a rush causes us to fuel our bodies in an unhealthy way, which then creates a downward spiral. The thoughts that go round and round in our head are most likely: 'Oh I'll be good tomorrow . . .' 'I'm just so tired I can't be bothered to cook, let's grab a take-out . . .' 'I'm starving, I haven't eaten all day apart from a coffee and chocolate at 3pm to keep me going.'

Not eating balanced meals during the day sets your blood sugar levels all over the place, resulting in cravings and energy lows, which is why you find yourself reaching for a refined carb option and sugar-laden treats by the afternoon.

Two years ago I was training chefs in a production kitchen away from home and for two months I was just seeing the inside of my hotel room and the inside of the kitchen. You might think I was cooking healthy food all day, but when I am cooking I tend not to be hungry until about two hours after I finish. I was so tired by then that I just found myself ordering off the hotel menu, asking for things I would never usually choose like pizza and pasta, because I wanted 'comfort food'. I was also too tired to exercise in the mornings. About five weeks into this stint I realised that I needed to snap out of it. I started doing just 20 minutes HIIT workouts (High Intensity Interval Training) in my room with no equipment before going to work. When I got to work, I made myself a massive bottle of green smoothie and sipped it throughout the morning, and then before leaving I grabbed some roasted vegetables, some seeds and a dressing and took them back with me to the hotel to have when I got hungry. Within three days I was bouncing off the walls again with energy, which made me realise that *it takes such little effort to give you an abundance of energy*. When I added it up, the only extra time I was using of my day was 35 minutes, and that included my exercise plan and preparing breakfast and dinner.

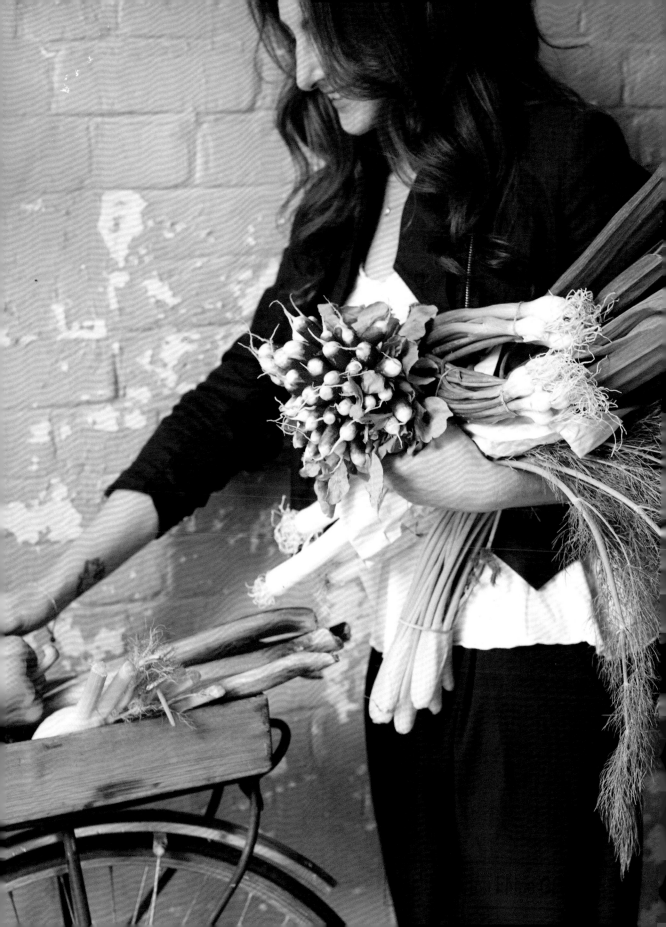

how to cook healthy in a hurry

This book is designed for you to cook in three different ways that take little time: QUICK, QUICK QUICK SLOW and COOK ONCE EAT TWICE. There are also BASIC recipes for a few store-cupboard staples. Each category has an icon (see below). Each recipe has one (or sometimes two) of the icons, so you can easily flick through and match the time you have available to the recipes you want to cook, pick out a recipe that you can cook in advance on a prep night, or look up a basic recipe for nut milk, bread or just a tasty salad.

QUICK These are the straightforward recipes that take less than 30 minutes.

QUICK QUICK SLOW These are recipes, such as cakes and bakes, that are quick to bring together and don't need much prep time from you, but then take a longer time in the oven, which you don't need to be in the kitchen for.

1+2

COOK ONCE EAT TWICE These are the recipes that take advantage of food you've prepared in advance. For example, if you cook a batch of vegetables and some grains and pulses at the weekend, you will be able to make several of these recipes from them during the course of your week.

BASIC recipes are my home-made nutritious versions of everyday items you might once have popped in your shopping basket. Making your own non-dairy milk, stock, bread, jam and pesto will save you time and tend to be much healthier than ready-made versions, plus they taste fantastic.

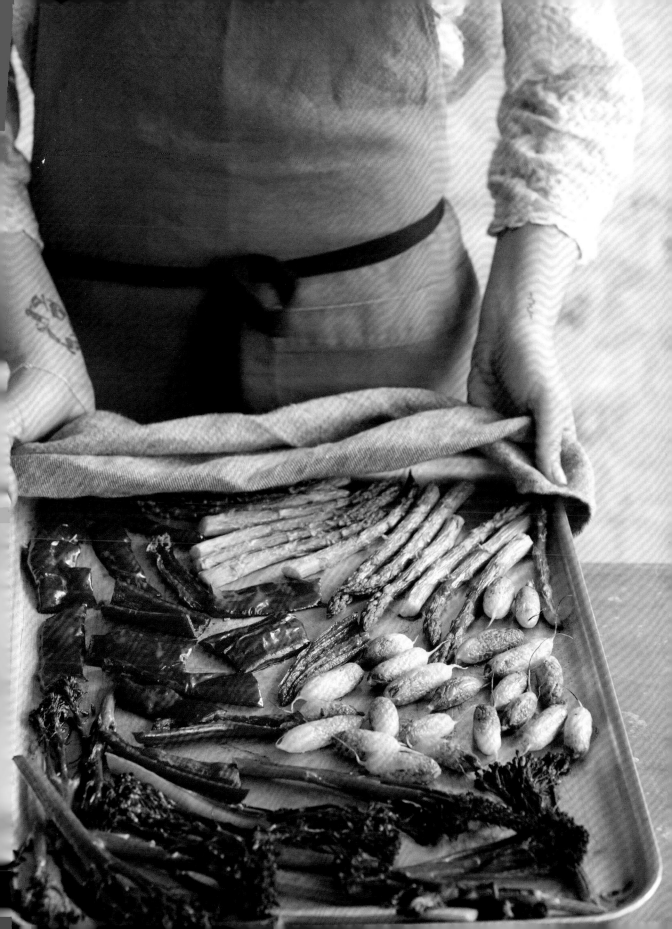

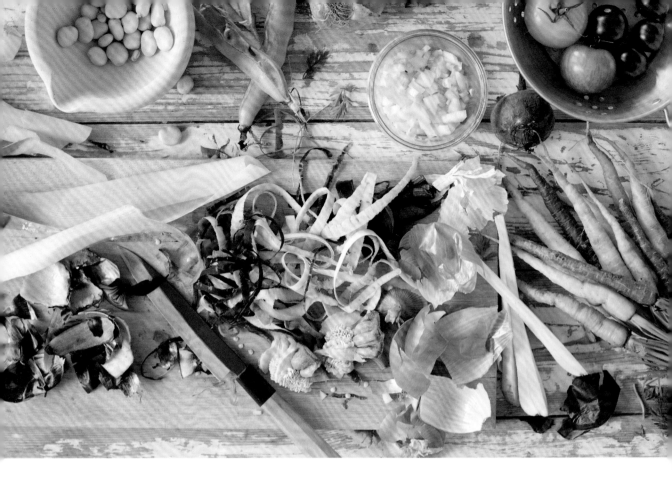

sunday prep night

Preparing your food ahead is key. Sunday night is my prep night and throughout the book you will see recipes that show you how you can make many different meals using your prep night veg. On a Sunday I will roast about three different trays of vegetables, cook some grains and pulses, make two salad dressings, wash my greens and make a dip for the week. That way it doesn't matter how tired I get, I will always have food in my fridge that I can pull together in a few minutes.

Batch cooking and freezing is the most cost-effective way to cook and eat. I love to make large curries, soups, cakes and treats and freeze them in single-portion freezer bags so they can be heated up from frozen with absolutely no fuss.

Finding time to do advance food prep is half the battle. If you can book it into your diary like a meeting or a date with a friend, then it's always there and, no matter what, it doesn't get moved. I have a few of these appointments in my diary. And along with my prep cooking there is my gym time and one night a week when it is time for me to watch a movie, take a bath uninterrupted, treat myself to a massage or just go for a walk. Whatever happens, those dates with myself don't get cancelled for anything!

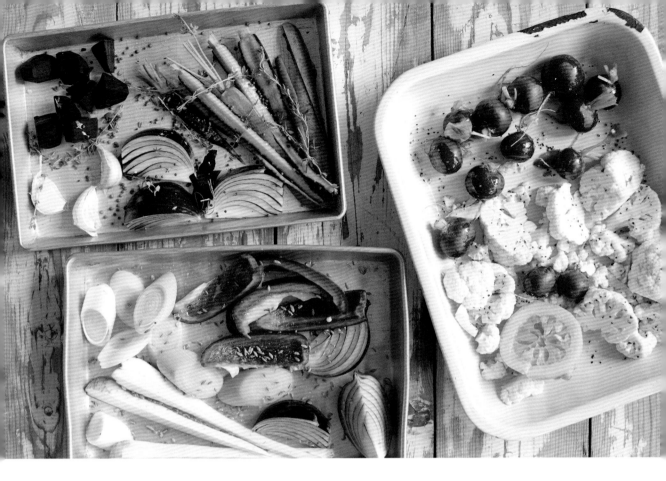

batch cooking for the whole family

Getting the whole family engaged in being healthy is so important to me. I love going over to my sister's house and cooking with the kids, as they love getting involved. Being healthy for yourself doesn't mean that you have to cook twice: with small alterations before serving you can create healthy meals for the whole family.

Roasted sweet potatoes, for example, can be used for both adults and kids in recipes like the Root vegetable, quinoa and feta cakes (see page 109) or Sweet potato falafels (see page 148). If you have little ones, you can also use the roasted sweet potato to blend into a purée for babies for weaning, stir it into mashed potato as a side dish, mix with pasta or rice noodles, make into pancakes or use as a topping for a pie.

Having frozen pesto (see page 181) in the freezer means you can use it for the kids and also make it into a delicious Spring minestrone soup (see page 70) for you.

Making batches of brownies or ice-cream keeps not only you off the refined sugar, but also the whole family. Just put into the freezer and grab when you need!

sunday night cooking

Roast vegetables

I suggest you roast two trays of vegetables on your prep night: hard root vegetables in one tray and soft vegetables in another.

Hard veg: sweet potato, butternut squash, aubergine, carrots, beetroot, celeriac, cauliflower, etc

Soft veg: courgettes, fennel, peppers, celery, onions, etc

Preheat the oven to 180°C/160°C fan/gas mark 4.

I always roast sweet potato and/or butternut squash on my prep nights. You can roast them whole, then cut in half and scoop out the flesh to add to a cake mix or purée. Alternatively, for adding to a salad, cut into wedges without peeling. To add to a hot dish, cut in half lengthways, then cut each half into 1cm half-moons or just roughly chop into 1cm chunks. I specify the best size in each recipe.

Your selection of aubergine, carrots, beetroot, celeriac and so forth can all be chopped and added to the baking tray with the sweet potato and squash.

Put together another tray of the chopped or whole soft vegetables too.

Drizzle the vegetables with sunflower oil, add a sprinkle of salt, then roast in the oven for 25–40 minutes until soft. The timings will vary depending on the vegetables you use and the size you cut them. Keep testing with a sharp knife until all the vegetables in the tray are just soft, then remove from the oven. Set aside to cool.

Cook grains:

Quinoa: This is cooked much like rice. Start by rinsing or soaking in water. Measure the quinoa into a saucepan with double the amount of water. Bring to the boil, then cover and simmer for about 15 minutes, or according to the packet instructions, until the germ separates from the seed. Rinse under freezing cold water until completely cool.

Brown rice: Measure the rice into a saucepan with two and a half times the amount of water. Bring to the boil, then cover and simmer for about 40–50 minutes, or according to the packet instructions until the rice is tender and the liquid has been absorbed. Rinse under freezing cold water and let stand for a few minutes before fluffing up with a fork.

Wild rice: Measure the rice into a saucepan with four times the amount of water. Bring to the boil, then cover and simmer for about 45–55 minutes, or according to the packet instructions, until the rice puffs open. Drain off the excess water and rinse under freezing cold water until completely cool.

Millet: Measure the millet into a saucepan with double the amount of water. Add a tablespoon of bouillon powder to give extra flavour and bring to the boil. Cover and simmer for about 20 minutes, or according to the packet instructions. When you take the millet off the heat, place in a sieve and make sure you soak it in freezing cold water as if you don't, it will be very gluey and sticky, not fluffy. Leave to drain.

You can watch my How to Cook Your Grains safely video on my YouTube channel Honestly Healthy.

Cook pulses:

Lentils: I like to use Puy lentils in my recipes as they taste wonderful and don't get mushy. To cook, rinse the lentils in cold water. Measure them into a saucepan with three times the amount of water and boil for 20–25 minutes, or according to the packet instructions (other types of lentil may need more or less cooking time). Drain.

Beans: Check the packet instructions carefully as some beans require overnight soaking. To cook, rinse the beans in cold water. Measure them into a saucepan with one and a half times the amount of water and boil for 30 minutes to 2 hours, topping up with more water if needed. The time will vary according to the variety of bean, so follow the packet instructions. You can also cook the beans with kombu seaweed to aid digestion when eating.

Make three salad dressings

Choose from the following delicious dressings:

Goat yoghurt dressing from the Middle Eastern potato salad (see page 78)

Coconut dressing from the Shiitake stir-fry (see page 96)

Tahini dressing from the Creamy tahini lentils with drippy boiled eggs (see page 104)

Miso dressing from the Griddled aubergine miso salad (see page 110) or Open nori sandwich with sweet potato butter (see page 150)

Parsley dressing from the Roasted radish and citrus salad (see page 120)

Pomegranate molasses dressing from the Rice, blackberry and carrot salad (see page 128)

Mint yoghurt dressing from the Warm halloumi and mint salad (see page 139)

Apple cider vinegar dressing from the Leek and halloumi millet salad (see page 138)

Ginger and lime dressing from the Asian noodle salad (see page 142)

Wash salads and leaves

Separate the leaves from any roots and wash under cold water. Using a salad spinner is the best way to dry the leaves, but you can also dry them in a tea towel. Wrap the washed leaves in kitchen paper and store in your fridge for 4–5 days. Alternatively, place them in an airtight container or your salad crisper box. You can now easily pull out a handful whenever needed.

Blanch green vegetables

Blanch your green vegetables in boiling salted water for just 3–4 minutes, until slightly softened, but still bright green. Run under freezing cold water straight away and drain. You can now keep the vegetables for 4–5 days in the fridge. You can watch my How to Blanch Your Greens video on my YouTube channel Honestly Healthy.

Batch cook and freeze

These recipes are great for batch cooking and freezing:

› Butternut, fennel and ginger soup (see page 66)

› Broccoli soup (see page 69)

› Curried aubergine (see page 94)

› Celeriac and polenta mash (see page 126)

Make a frittata with any leftovers

The Leftovers duck egg frittata (see page 102) shows you how to make a duck (or hen's) egg frittata. You don't have to stick to the vegetables I suggest – you really can use pretty much anything. Select something you have cooked on your prep night or use up any vegetables lurking in your fridge – just ensure you season as suggested.

Make a breakfast in advance

It's great to have at least one breakfast in the fridge so you can reach in and grab it on a busy morning. Try one of these recipes:

› Chia breakfast with blueberry compote (see page 44)

› Avocado 'yoghurt' breakfast (see page 38)

› Cacao granola (see page 50)

Hard-boiled eggs

Hard-boil your eggs in boiling salted water for 10 minutes. Place under cold running water to quickly cool, then remove from the water promptly so no bacteria can grow. Dry and store the eggs in their shells in the fridge for up to a week. Make sure you don't store next to any strong-smelling or -tasting foods as eggs can absorb flavours and odours.

Bake brownies or granola bars

When the oven is free, make your choice of bakes. Try one of these:

› Quinoa granola bars (see page 169)

› Cauliflower protein brownies (page 206)

checklist sunday night prep

You don't have to do everything listed below; even if you just pick a few, it will transform your week.

Roast vegetables

Cook grains: quinoa, brown/wild rice, millet

Cook pulses: lentils and beans

Make three salad dressings

Wash salads and leaves

Blanch green vegetables: broccoli, green beans, kale

Batch cook and freeze: soups, curry, stews

Make a frittata with any leftovers

Make a breakfast in advance

Hard-boil eggs for breakfasts, lunches and snacks

Bake brownies or granola bars for your sweet treat

prep night cooking guide

Opposite I've put together a list of my favourite vegetables, grains and pulses that I cook on prep night. I've added the uncooked and cooked weights so you can easily swap the cooked vegetables or grains into any recipe and cut the preparation time right down. There's also information about the cooking methods that I prefer using for each ingredient, the times and what size to cut the veggies so you can group similar types together in one tray.

	Uncooked weight	Roasted at 180°C	Blanched or boiled	Size when chopped	Amount of oil	Cooking time
Hard veg						
Aubergine	400g	180g	—	2cm square	1 tsp	20 mins
Beetroot	400g	230g	—	2cm square	1 tsp	40 mins
Butternut squash	400g	275g	—	2cm square	1 tsp	35 mins
Carrots	400g	240g	—	2cm square	1 tsp	45 mins
Celeriac	400g	290g	—	2cm square	1 tsp	45 mins
Sweet potato	400g	280g	—	2cm square	1 tsp	35 mins
Soft veg						
Asparagus	200g	150g	200g	whole	½ tsp	20 mins roasted/ 5 mins boiled
Beans	200g	—	200g	whole	—	3 mins
Broccoli	200g	140g	240g	medium florets	½ tsp	25 mins roasted/ 3 mins blanched
Cauliflower	400g	290g	410g	medium florets	1 tsp	25 mins roasted/ 10 mins steamed
Courgette	200g	165g	—	2cm thick slices	½ tsp	25 mins
Fennel	200g	150g	—	1 bulb in 6 pieces	½ tsp	30 mins
Frozen peas	200g	—	200g	—	—	2 mins
Red pepper	200g (1 whole pepper)	150g	—	1 pepper in 6 pieces	½ tsp	25 mins
Radishes	200g	150g	—	whole	½ tsp	10–15 mins depending on size
Grain and pulses						
Brown rice	100g	—	230g	—	—	45 mins
Chickpeas	100g	—	230g	—	—	50 mins
Millet	100g	—	240g	—	—	20 mins
Puy lentils	100g	—	230g	—	—	20 mins
Quinoa	100g	—	190g	—	—	20 mins

There are lots of brilliant healthy recipes out there, and once you have your prep night up and running, you'll want to experiment. Try my *Honestly Healthy* books or honestlyhealthyfood.com for more recipes.

how to put a simple prep night dinner together

Try these recipes from the book using your prep night cooking.

Cook in advance	Recipe
Roasted sweet potato	Sweet potato porridge (see page 32)
	Middle Eastern potato salad (see page 78)
	Ten-minute turmeric quinoa risotto (see page 86)
	Root vegetable, quinoa and feta cakes (see page 109)
	Herbed sweet potato salad (see page 130)
	Sweet potato falafels (see page 148)
Roasted butternut squash	Tagine and cauli couscous (see page 85)
	Root vegetable, quinoa and feta cakes (see page 109)
	Butternut squash and thyme salad (see page 153)
Roasted hard vegetables (cauliflower/beetroot/celeriac)	Roasted cauliflower and green bean sweet salad (see page 91)
	Beetroot and rosemary stew (see page 106)
	Cauliflower protein brownies (see page 206)
Precooked quinoa	Ten-minute turmeric quinoa risotto (see page 86)
	Root vegetable, quinoa and feta cakes (see page 109)
	Griddled aubergine miso salad (see page 110)
Precooked millet	Leek and halloumi millet salad (see page 138)
Cooked wild/brown rice	Roasted radish and citrus salad (see page 120)
	Rice, blackberry and carrot salad (see page 128)
Cooked lentils	Creamy tahini lentils with drippy boiled eggs (see page 104)
	Beetroot burgers (see page 116)
Hard-boiled eggs	Smashed eggs and avocado (see page 36)
	Cucumber noodle asparagus broth (see page 74)
	Creamy tahini lentils with drippy boiled eggs (see page 104)

three great
dishes from
your prep night
sweet potato

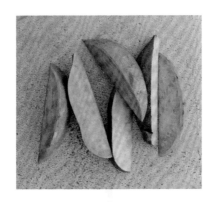

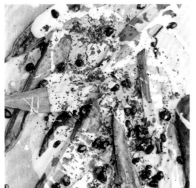

page 78

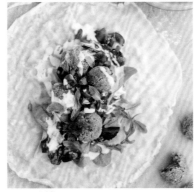

page 148

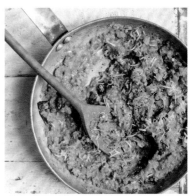

page 86

three great
dishes from
your prep night
cauliflower

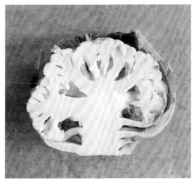

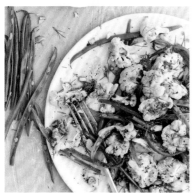

page 91

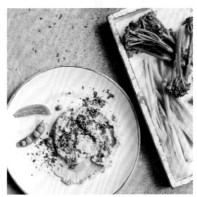

page 184

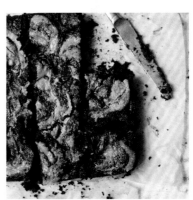

page 206

great flavour combos for your prep night veg

These recipes give some great ideas, but you don't have to follow a recipe to the letter to make a delicious prep night dinner. Take the chance to experiment and substitute any of the vegetables for whatever is in season. If you follow the prep list, you will have plenty of combinations to put together. I always say if you have the same salad every day with a different dressing, it will taste like a different dish. Here are some great flavour combos:

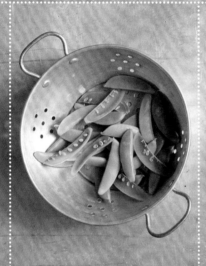
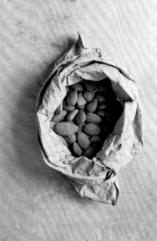
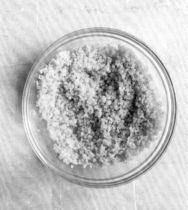

Vegetable	Pulse/ Protein	Grain
Roasted sweet potato	Puy lentils	—
Rosted/steamed butternut squash	Flaked almonds	Quinoa
Roasted pepper	Edamame beans	Millet
Roasted sweet potato	Tempeh or tofu	Brown rice
Blanched broccoli/peas	Sesame seeds	Wild rice or quinoa
Roasted aubergine	Chickpeas	—

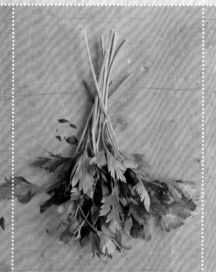
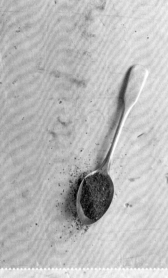
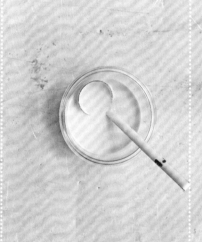

Herb	Spice	Dressing
Parsley	Cumin seeds	Goats' milk yoghurt and a pinch of ground cumin, cinnamon and salt
Coriander	Ground coriander	Lemon, olive oil and salt
Dill	Fennel seeds	Brown rice vinegar, salt and lemon
Parsley	Cumin seeds	Tamari and olive oil
Dill	Sumac	Yoghurt, salt, lemon and garlic
Coriander	Ground cinnamon	Sweet miso dressing

time-saving tips

1. Buy your larder ingredients online so you never have to lug them back from the supermarket again.

2. Make your own stock cubes and freeze them (page 118). This saves time chopping and weighing out ingredients to start off the base of a dish.

3. Make and freeze pesto in ice cubes (page 181). Chuck them into soups, pasta or stir-fries for instant flavour.

4. Wash and chop fresh fruit and store in freezer bags. Defrost for quick smoothies or as a topping for your porridge. You can watch my How Should You Freeze Your Fruit video on my YouTube channel Honestly Healthy.

5. Make and freeze soup or stews.

6. Plan your meals ahead for the week to save money. You can download my free seven-day meal planner from my website *honestlyhealthyfood.com*

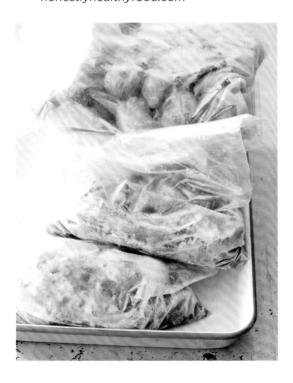

healthy swaps

Magazines, newspapers and the internet are full of recipes that you might like to try and remember if a recipe lists any of the following, try just substituting with some of my healthy alternative swaps. For example if a recipe calls for white bread, you can upgrade to gluten-free, millet or rice bread to make your dish more healthy.

Ingredient	Substitution
White bread	Gluten-free, millet or rice bread
Cows' milk	Almond, rice, coconut or any other plant milk
Cows' milk yoghurt	Soya, goats' milk or sheeps' milk yoghurt
Sugar	Coconut palm sugar, rice syrup, coconut blossom syrup, agave
Cornflour	Kuzu for thickening
Wheat flour	Gluten-free rice, buckwheat or teff flour
Coffee	Instant barley coffee

healthy travelling

A lot of people ask me how do I stay healthy when travelling? Again, it comes down to preparation. If I'm taking an early flight, I will put the ingredients for a green smoothie in the blender the night before, but I won't blend them until the morning. I then put the smoothie into a bottle and swig it on the way to the airport.

You can also make a thick bircher muesli to take with you or a simple frittata or roasted vegetables with quinoa mixed through with hummus, and some granola bars for snacks. They'll all get through security – all it takes is a little planning.

No more soggy salads!

Cover a teacup or ramekin with clingfilm and pour in your salad dressing. Twist tightly to seal and place on top of your salad in a screwtop jar or airtight plastic container. Your salad is now ready to dress whenever you're ready to eat. I have a step by step tutorial on my YouTube channel.

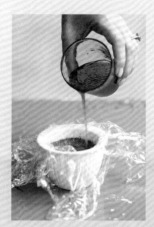
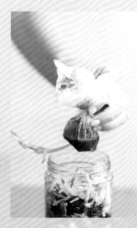
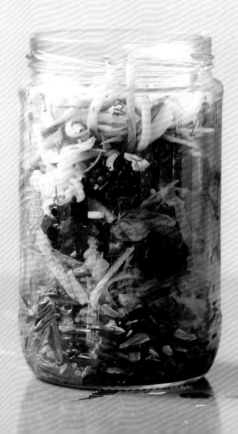

glossary of ingredients

Agar flakes – Made from seaweed, these vegan flakes can be used instead of gelatine to set a mousse or jelly. They are very alkaline and therefore great for digestion.

Agave powder and syrup – Also known as agave nectar, this sweetener is derived from the blue weber agave plant and is sweeter than refined sugar. Always buy organic raw agave and use it in small quantities. It has a low glycaemic index, so doesn't cause swings in blood sugar levels.

Alkaline greens powder – A great supplement to add to a smoothie to make your body more alkaline and boost your nutritional intake.

Apple cider vinegar – The only alkaline vinegar, this condiment is made from fermented apple cider.

Arame seaweed – Sold in packs of dried strips, arame has a slightly sweet and delicate flavour and is almost black in colour.

Baobab powder – The fruit of the baobab is dried on the tree, harvested and then ground into a powder. This tangy powder is more potent than vitamin C and helps to keep you well year round.

Barley coffee – In the past this naturally caffeine-free version of coffee was drunk by Italian peasants as they couldn't afford the real thing. It's sold as a powder that's mixed with hot water and perks you up.

Bee pollen – This granular garnish is made by worker bees, who pack pollen into little granules with added honey or nectar. Sold in small jars, a little goes a long way; it's highly nutritious and adds great texture to salads and smoothies.

Bouillon powder – This vegetarian instant stock powder is made only from vegetables and is free from preservatives, GM organisms, artificial flavours and colours.

Brown rice miso – Rice miso is made by fermenting soya beans with salt and a fungus and adding rice. The brown rice version is a modern addition to traditional miso pastes as only recently have we learnt how to ferment unpolished rice. Miso is high in protein and rich in vitamins and minerals.

Brown rice vinegar – A delicious Japanese condiment, this is slightly sweet and doesn't have the acidity of other vinegars.

Chia seeds – Grown as a grain, originally in Mexico and Guatemala, these seeds are a rich source of energy. They have the highest level of omega-3 fatty acids of any seed and can absorb up to 15 times their own weight in fluid, so make a great thickening agent. Available in both black and white, chia seeds are nutritionally similar, but the colour of the white seeds means they disappear more easily into food.

Coconut blossom syrup – This sweetener has a low glycaemic index, so keeps blood sugar levels balanced. If you can't find it, substitute it with agave syrup.

Coconut oil – I have switched to coconut oil in most of my cooking as it is packed with beneficial fatty acids. Look for raw, cold-pressed (sometimes labelled extra virgin) oil to be sure it is free of chemicals. Coconut oil is solid at room temperature, so can be used instead of butter or margarine, or heated to form a liquid.

Coconut palm sugar – More nutritious than ordinary sugar but just as sweet, palm sugar is made from the sap of the coconut palm tree. It has a low glycaemic index but use it in small amounts to avoid getting hooked on its sweetness. Look for organic and unprocessed versions, and check it's a pure coconut palm product.

Date syrup – A natural sweetener made from just puréed dates.

Himalayan pink salt – A rose-coloured salt mined in the foothills of the Himalayan Mountains, this is an ancient product first created thousands of years ago. It's high in iron, potassium and magnesium, which are all vital for good health.

Lucuma powder – The dried powder of the lucuma fruit from South America adds a certain maple syrup sweetness to foods or drinks. It also helps to maintain blood sugar levels as it has a low glycaemic index. It's naturally rich in vitamins, protein and zinc.

Maca powder – Also known as Peruvian ginseng, maca powder has been used in Peru for endurance and energy for over 2000 years. It adds a certain malty sweetness to smoothies and desserts.

Matcha powder – This green powder, sold in small tins, is made from green tea leaves that have been ground very finely. Traditionally drunk in Japan as part of the tea ceremony and by monks, matcha promotes alertness and focus. It imparts a pleasing green colour and has a slightly bitter taste.

Mirin – This essential condiment used in Japanese cooking is a sweetened sake or rice wine with a light syrupy texture. It offers a wonderfully mild sweetness to dishes.

Miso – *see* Brown rice miso and Sweet miso

Nori seaweed – Produced in sheets, nori is available toasted or untoasted, and is used for wrapping sushi or eating as a snack. It can be deep green or purplish in colour and, as with all sea vegetables, is highly alkaline and full of amino acids.

Nutritional yeast – Sold in tubs as flakes, this ingredient is made from a single-celled yeast, *Saccharomyces cerevisiae*, which is grown on molasses, then harvested, washed and dried with heat to 'deactivate' it. So, unlike yeast for making bread, it has no leavening ability. A sprinkle of these flakes packs a nutritional punch and adds a certain savouriness to lots of dishes.

Puffed quinoa – Also called quinoa pops, these are simply popped quinoa seeds. Buy from a health food shop or pop your own in a hot dry pan.

Quinoa flakes – These are essentially raw quinoa seeds that have been rolled flat to create thin flakes. Nutrient-rich and gluten-free, they're fast-cooking, due to their thinness.

Raw cacao butter – A butter rich in nutrients that can be used to make raw chocolate, cakes and puddings.

Raw cacao powder – Unlike normal cocoa powder, raw cacao powder is made from unroasted beans, which means it retains more of its nutrients and antioxidants.

Sprouts – Anyone can sprout seeds or beans on a windowsill or in a plant pot. These nutritious and delicious micro-greens come in as many kinds as there are seeds or beans. Popular ones include aduki bean, alfalfa, broccoli, mustard and cress, mung bean and rose sprouts.

Sumac – This tangy, lemony spice is often used in Mediterranean and Middle Eastern cooking. It's made from the berries of *Rhus coriaria*, which are bright red, so it has a vibrant colour too.

Sweet miso – Historically this condiment was the preserve of the rich because it is made with lots of rice koji (mould spores), which in the past were very expensive. This type of miso has a wonderful creamy richness and slightly salty sweetness.

Tahini – A thick paste made from ground sesame seeds, tahini is often used in Middle Eastern cooking. It packs a high-protein punch and is wonderfully versatile – it can be used in baking or dressings, for instance. It has a lovely nutty flavour.

Tamari – Essentially a wheat-free soy sauce, tamari can be used if you need to make a dish gluten-free. Its taste does differ slightly from regular soy sauce – it's less salty – and has a dark, rich colour, but can be used in the same way.

Turmeric – Quite a different thing from the ground version, fresh turmeric looks a bit like root ginger or a thin Jerusalem artichoke. Its flesh is bright orange (watch out as it stains). It has an earthy, citrusy taste; and slight tongue-numbing qualities (rather like Sichuan pepper).

Vegan butter – This dairy-free spread is a mixture of oils that has a rich, buttery taste. It's available in tubs and can be used in just the same way as butter.

Vegan protein powder – I exercise a lot so a shake with added protein powder is part of my daily routine, aiding recovery and muscle and strength gain. Look for a vegan powder if you are following an alkaline diet, and check for added ingredients and sweeteners.

Xanthan gum – This ingredient keeps your home baking gluten-free. It's made by fermenting sugar with the bacterium *Xanthomonas campestris* and is available in a powdered form. It can be used as a thickening agent.

start
the
day

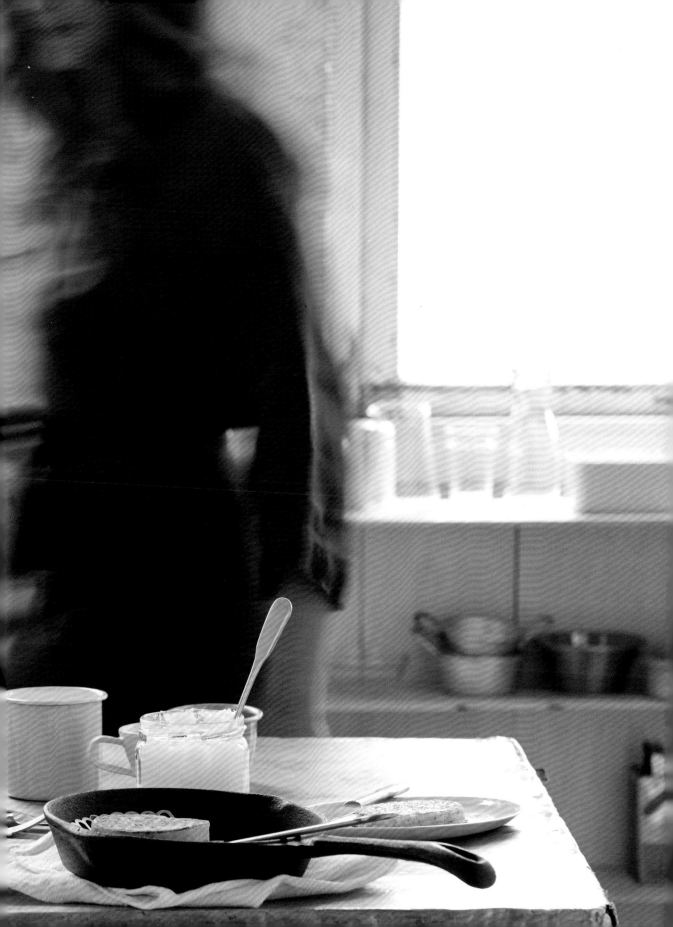

Drinking a green smoothie is the best way to start your morning – they have so much goodness to kick-start you. I love to throw anything in them to set me up for the day. It's a great breakfast you can take to work that only takes a couple of minutes to blend together.

SERVES 2

Matcha is a really flavoursome green tea powder and provides the body with a fantastic energy kick. It's also really high in antioxidants so makes the perfect addition to a smoothie. I love the gentle flavours of this recipe and if you want to turn it into an ice-cold number, just add a handful of ice to the blender as you blitz. Add a few more dates too if you would like it a little sweeter. You can make this without the matcha and you get a slightly paler smoothie.

SERVES 1–2

green apricot smoothie

matcha avocado smoothie

2 fresh apricots, stones removed
¼ avocado, peeled and stone removed
5cm piece of cucumber
large handful of spinach
½ tsp alkaline greens powder
1 date (optional)
½ banana
125ml almond milk (bought or see page 52)

Place all of the ingredients in a blender with 250ml water and blitz until smooth. Add a couple of ice cubes too to make it extra cold. Drink straight away.

1 avocado, peeled and stone removed
130g melon, peeled and chopped
185ml almond or other plant milk (bought or see page 52)
¼ tsp vanilla extract
3 dates
¼ tsp matcha powder

Put all of the ingredients into a blender with 315ml water and blitz until velvety smooth. Drink straight away.

From left to right: green apricot smoothie; avocado smoothie; matcha avocado smoothie.

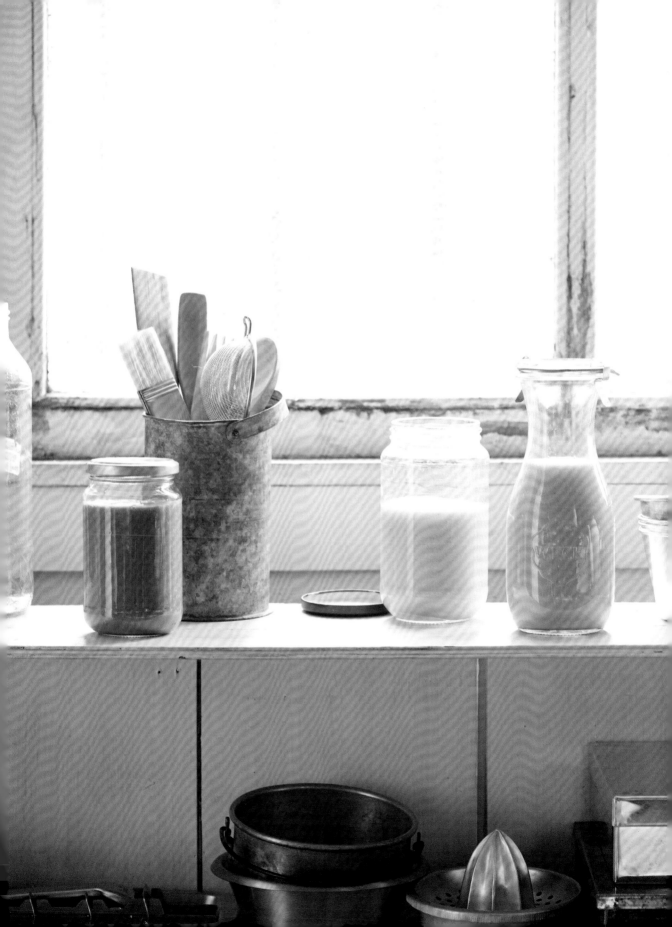

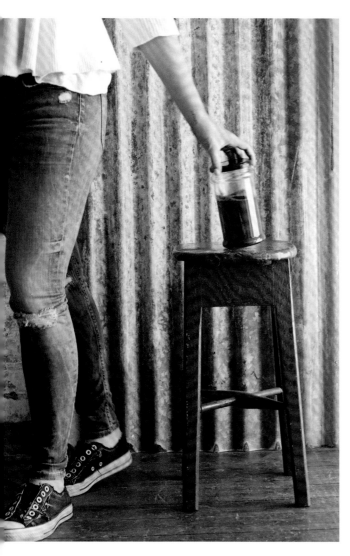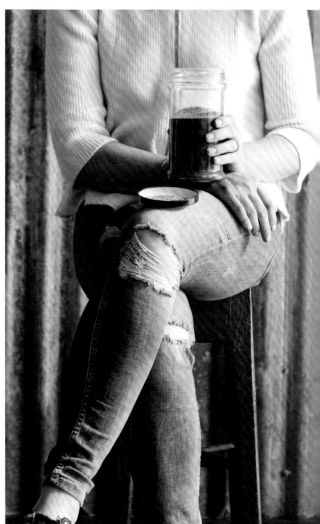

Beetroot is a fantastic ingredient to use in your smoothies and shakes if you are working out a lot. Naturally occurring nitrates ensure that more oxygenated blood is carried to the muscles, which essentially allows for better endurance. Perfect for any runners out there. I work out a lot and a daily protein shake is key to my routine (see photo opposite).

SERVES 1

Grapefruit is, surprisingly, one of the most alkaline fruits you can have, so it's a great one to start the day. The mellow flavours of cucumber and celery make this a wonderfully hydrating juice. Blitz up with ice and make a simple sorbet with any leftovers! (see photo on page 31)

SERVES 1

strawberry and beetroot protein shake

grapefruit, cucumber and celery juice

190g strawberries
2 tbsp vegan protein powder
100g sheeps' milk or coconut yoghurt
¼ tsp vanilla extract
60g beetroot, peeled and roughly chopped (or grated if you do not have a powerful blender)
2 tbsp cashew butter
handful of ice (optional)

Put all of the ingredients into a high-speed blender with 125ml water and blitz until velvety smooth. If you want to serve it nice and cold, add the ice for that extra cooling blast.

115g cucumber, peeled
1 whole pink grapefruit, peeled
2 sticks celery
50g strawberries

Press all of the ingredients through a juicer, adding 125ml water at the end to flush out any remaining bits.

Serve as it is or put the juice into a blender with lots of ice and blitz to make a super-refreshing slushie.

Both apple cider vinegar and ginger are known to be fantastic for the digestion. They can be a little sharp on their own so I like to blend them into green juices. When it comes to juices and smoothies, the more veg the better, and every now and then I think it is really good to opt for an entirely vegetable-based juice or smoothie. And if you can make all of the ingredients green, so much the better. The ingredients in this juice are incredibly alkaline, so if you can work a juice like this into your weekly routine, you will be doing your body the world of good.

SERVES 1

All of the ingredients in this juice are incredibly cleansing, so this is my go-to juice if I am ever feeling bloated and a little lethargic. It is also packed with vitamin C, so works brilliantly if you are feeling a little under the weather.

SERVES 1

a green juice for digestion

fennel, pear and cucumber juice

170g courgettes
150g (roughly 2 sticks) celery
100g broccoli
35g parsley, stalks included
15g piece of root ginger
½ tsp apple cider vinegar

Press the courgettes, celery, broccoli, parsley and ginger through a juicer. While the juicer is on, pour in 60ml water to flush out any remnants of juice. Stir the apple cider vinegar through the juice and drink straight away if possible.

1 pear, peeled
270g (1 large) fennel, quartered
10cm (110g) piece of cucumber, peeled
juice of ¼ lime

Push the pear, fennel and cucumber through a juicer and then, while the juicer is still on, pour in 60ml water to flush out any remnants of juice. Stir in the lime juice and serve nice and cold.

From left to right: grapefruit, cucumber and celery juice; fennel, pear and cucumber juice; green juice for digestion.

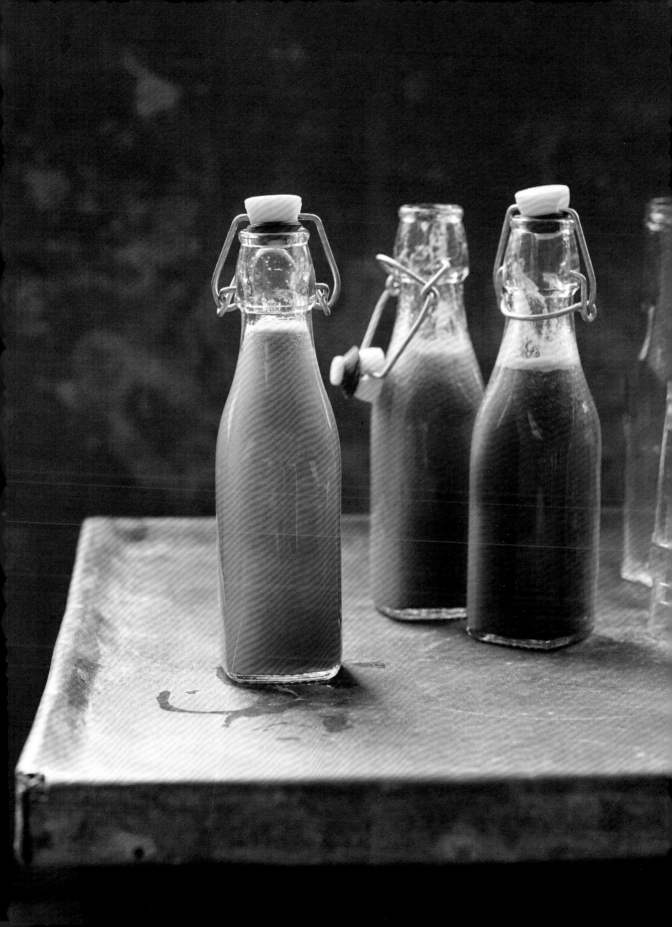

This is a wonderfully filling and nourishing quick breakfast that
you can make with leftover roast potatoes too. A great healthy energy
giver, it is perfect for a post-workout meal.

SERVES 2

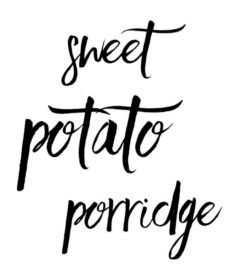

sweet potato porridge

Mash the flesh of the roasted sweet potato with a fork.

In a saucepan, add the sweet potato mash, oats, grated carrots, almond milk, cinnamon and 275ml water and cook over a medium to high heat for 4 minutes.

Stir in the coconut oil and serve for a warming breakfast.

The porridge is naturally quite sweet, but if you would like that extra little edge of sweetness, add the agave syrup (date or coconut blossom syrup would also be delicious).

Garnish with blueberries, a dusting of cinnamon and agave if you wish.

85g roasted sweet potato (125g raw sweet potato, roasted whole) (see page 12)
65g oats
35g carrots, grated
100ml almond or other plant milk (bought or see page 52)
½ tsp ground cinnamon
1 tsp coconut oil
1 tbsp agave syrup (optional)

for the garnish (optional)
blueberries, sliced
ground cinnamon
agave syrup, to garnish

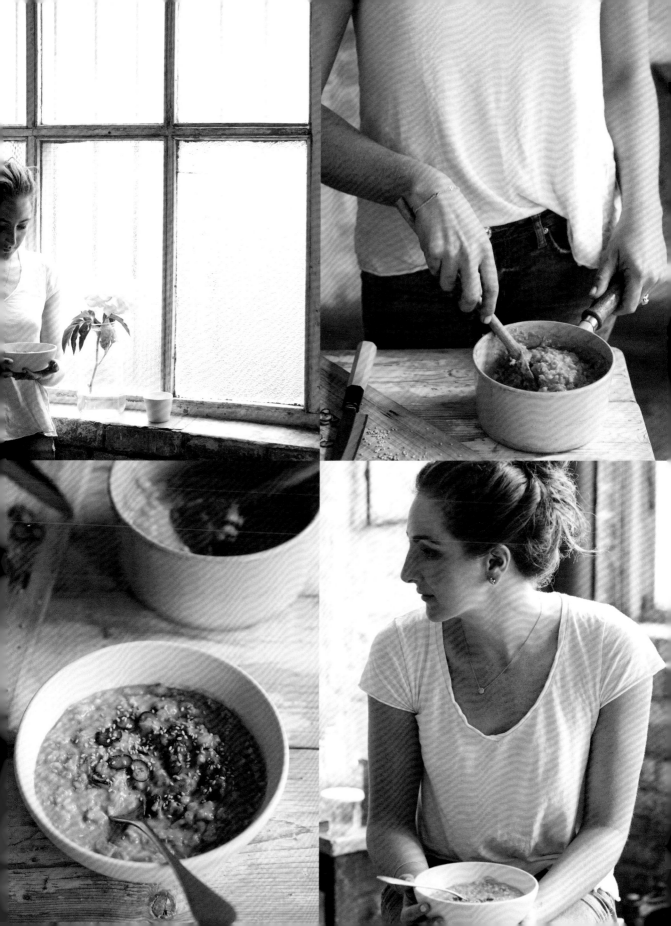

A wonderfully warming and nourishing porridge to start the day and such a lovely alternative to normal oats. Teff has become a huge part of my cooking as it is so nutrient dense and a wonderful grain to work with. Try adding different compotes over the top as well. You could even use the leftovers to make granola bars by adding some oats and dates to the mixture.

SERVES 2

teff *and* rhubarb porridge

Add the teff, almond milk and cinnamon to a pan and cook over a medium heat for 15 minutes, stirring regularly.

Add the oats and compote and mix for another 2–3 minutes until all of the liquid has been absorbed. If you need to loosen it up a little more, add a splash of almond milk.

To serve, add the extra compote, yoghurt and a sprinkle of bee pollen.

100g teff flour
360ml almond milk (bought or see page 52)
¼ tsp ground cinnamon
30g oats
120g Rhubarb compote (see page 197), plus 2 tbsp to serve

to serve:
4 tbsp yoghurt
a sprinkling of bee pollen

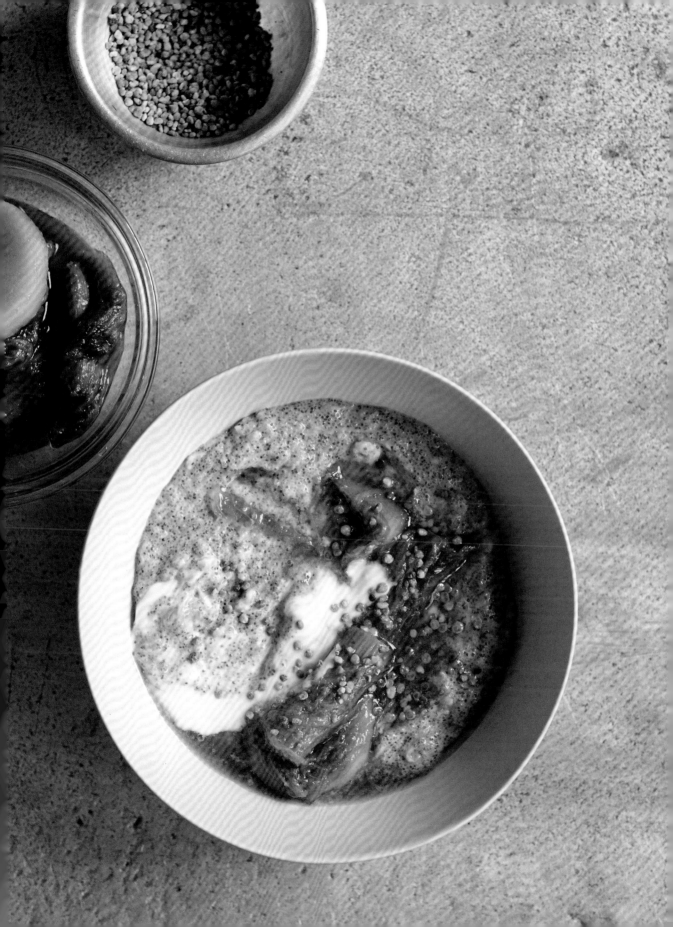

This is one step on from simple avocado on toast. Smashed-up boiled eggs take me back to my childhood. I always tend to boil up eggs on my prep night, so I have something on hand for a really quick but tasty breakfast.

SERVES 2

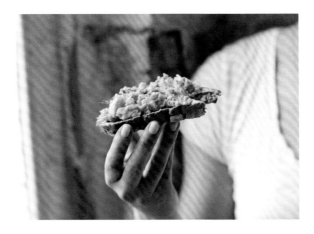

smashed eggs
and
avocado

Peel the boiled eggs and mash up with a fork. Chop the avocado, add this in and mash together. Add the lemon juice, a pinch of sumac, salt and pepper and mix.

Toast some gluten-free bread, butter with coconut oil and place the mixture evenly over the top.

Garnish with some fresh dill, if you like.

3 hard-boiled eggs (see page 14)
½ avocado
juice of ½ lemon
a pinch of sumac
a pinch of Himalayan pink salt
a pinch of freshly ground black pepper
2 slices gluten-free bread
coconut oil, for buttering toast
fresh dill, to garnish (optional)

❯ 1+2

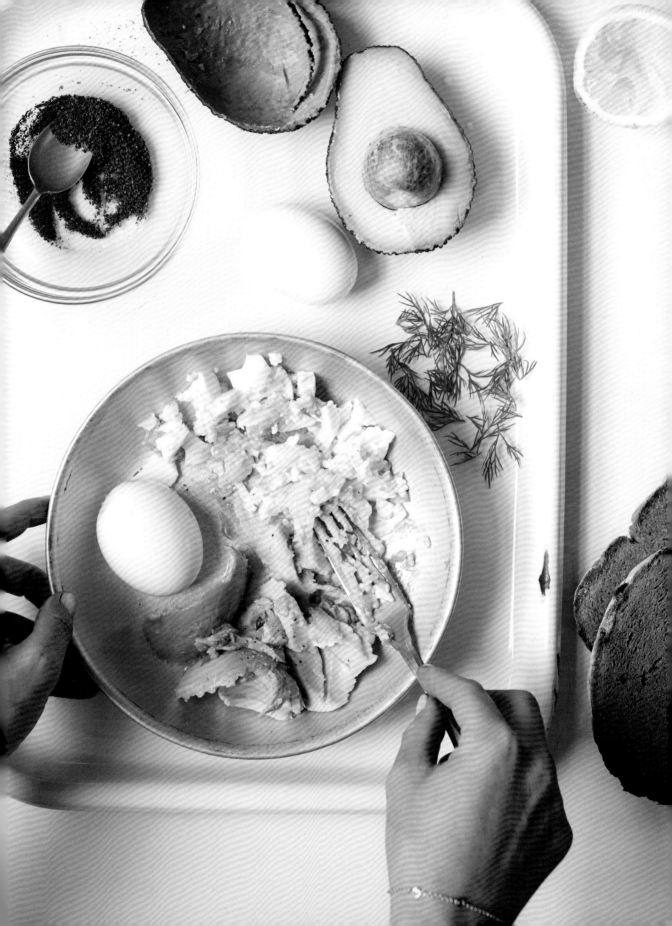

Not just for adults! This is a great sweet alternative to yoghurt, but is also wonderful for babies and kids to get them to eat more greens. The banana in this is so delicious. You can add your own fruit combinations and toppings – try home-made granola or mixed nuts and seeds.

SERVES 2

avocado 'yoghurt' breakfast

To make the avocado 'yoghurt', place all of the ingredients in a blender and blitz until velvety smooth. Transfer to two jars, bowls or plates and top with the mango, blackberries, cinnamon, seeds, granola (if using) and/or any other toppings.

Serve fresh or store in the fridge for up to 2 or 3 days for a quick on-the-go breakfast.

1 avocado, peeled and stone removed
½ banana
juice of ½ lemon
3 tbsp almond or other plant milk (bought or see page 52)

for the toppings:
80g mango, peeled and sliced
40g blackberries
a pinch of ground cinnamon
a sprinkle of mixed seeds
Cacao granola (see page 50) (optional)

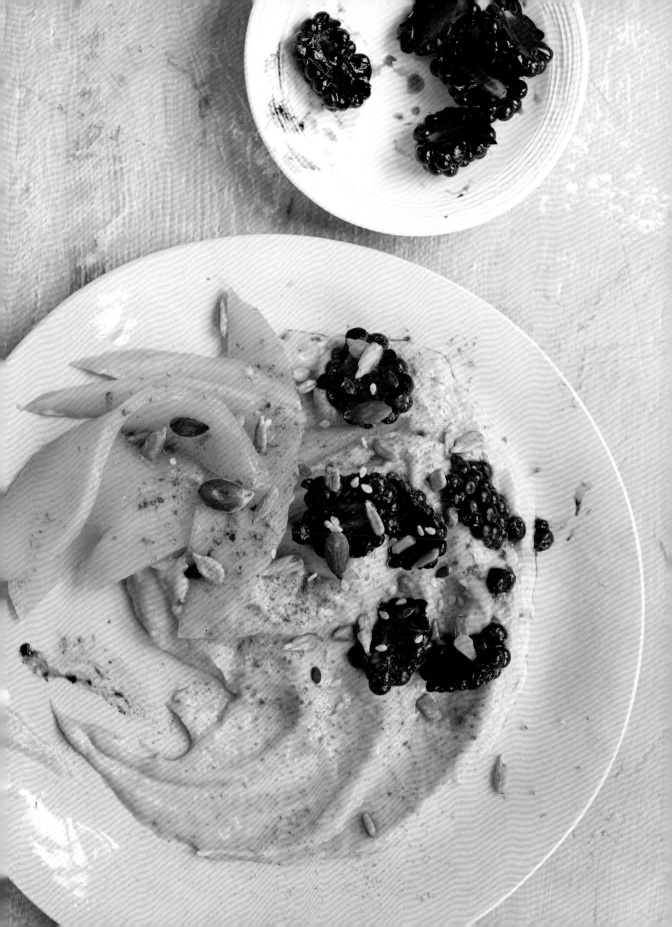

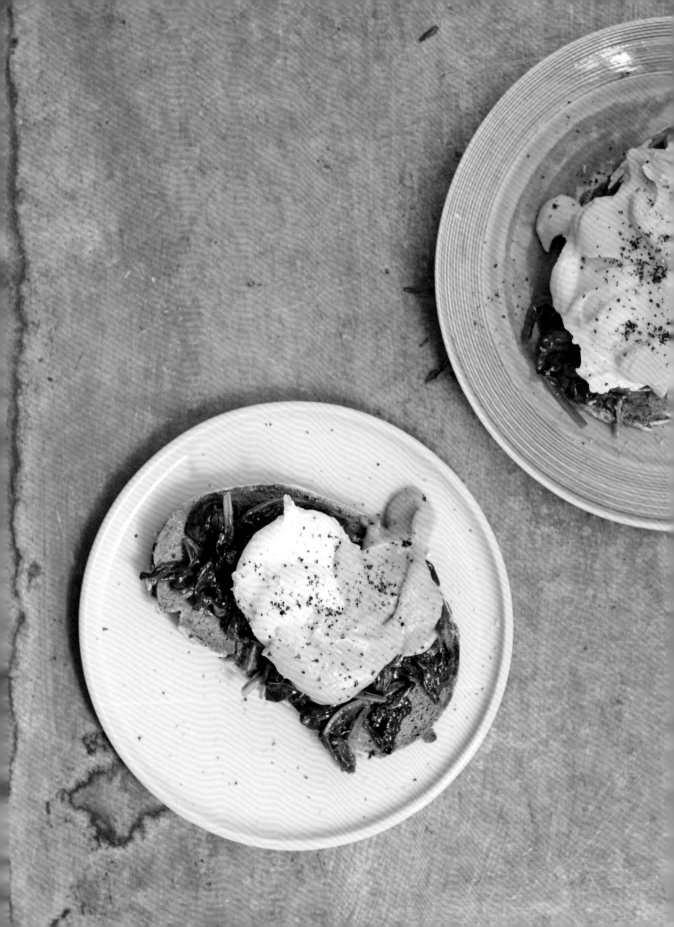

There is nothing better in my book than eggs and avocado on toast, so I have re-created it here to jazz up your mornings. If you don't eat eggs, you can just have this delicious avocado cream on toast by itself. Breakfast in bed is taken to a whole new level with this creation.

SERVES 2

creamed avocado AND poached eggs on toast

1 avocado, peeled and stone removed

juice of ½ lemon

60ml unsweetened rice milk

a pinch of Himalayan pink salt

a pinch of freshly ground black pepper

⅛ tsp apple cider vinegar

4 eggs

4 slices gluten-free bread

coconut oil, for buttering toast

wilted spinach (optional)

coriander leaves and a pinch of sumac, to garnish (optional)

Put the avocado into a blender, add the lemon juice, rice milk, vinegar, salt and pepper and blend till smooth.

Poach your eggs in boiling water with the cider vinegar and toast your bread.

To assemble, butter the toast with the coconut oil, cover with the spinach (if using), then the poached eggs and spoon over the avocado cream.

Garnish with fresh coriander leaves and a pinch of sumac if you like.

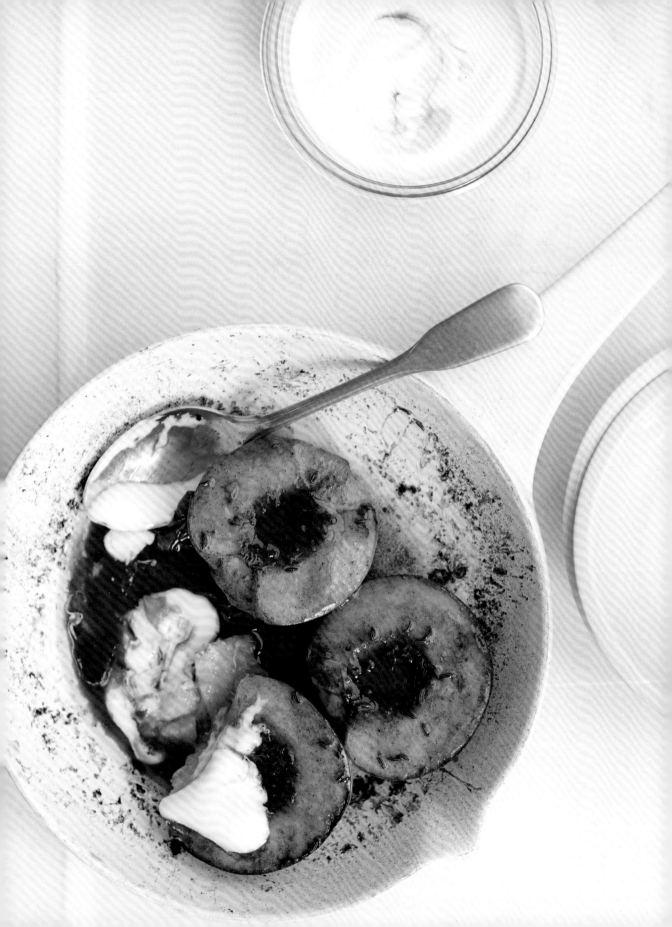

This is a really fresh and delicious alternative to stewed fruits.
There is little better than sweet peaches in the summer and
with a pinch of cinnamon, they make the best breakfast or dessert.
If you don't have caraway seeds, try fennel seeds – and if you don't
have either, don't worry, it will taste delicious anyway.

SERVES 2

warm peaches AND cinnamon drizzle

1 tbsp coconut oil
½ tsp ground cinnamon
a pinch of caraway seeds
¼ tsp vanilla extract
2 peaches, cut in half and
    stones removed
yoghurt, to serve

Melt the coconut oil in a heavy-bottomed frying pan and then add the cinnamon, caraway seeds, vanilla and 60ml water.

Add the peaches to the steaming pan and continue to heat for 3–5 minutes until the peaches are beginning to soften and brown. Add another 60ml water and continue to heat for a further 2–4 minutes.

Once the sauce is nice and thick and the peaches soft, remove from the heat and serve with a dollop of yoghurt.

You either love or hate chia – it's one of those acquired tastes because of the texture. However, this dish is gorgeous as it also has the wonderful, gentle soothing taste of star anise. This recipe is perfect for making on a Sunday prep night and having in the fridge for the rest of the week.

SERVES 4

chia breakfast with blueberry compote

Combine all of the ingredients for the 'porridge' in a bowl and whisk together with a fork. Leave to sit for a couple of minutes before whisking again so as to remove any 'clumps' of seeds that may have formed. Refrigerate overnight or for 6 hours.

To make the compote, bring all the ingredients to a gentle simmer with 120ml water in a small saucepan and continue to heat for 5–6 minutes until the blueberries soften.

Serve the 'porridge' and compote together.

50g white chia seeds
300ml almond or other plant milk (bought or see page 52)
2 star anise
¼ tsp vanilla extract
½ tsp coconut blossom syrup
½ tsp lucuma powder

for the blueberry compote:
200g frozen blueberries
4 star anise
4 tsp agave syrup
zest of 1 lemon
2 tbsp tahini

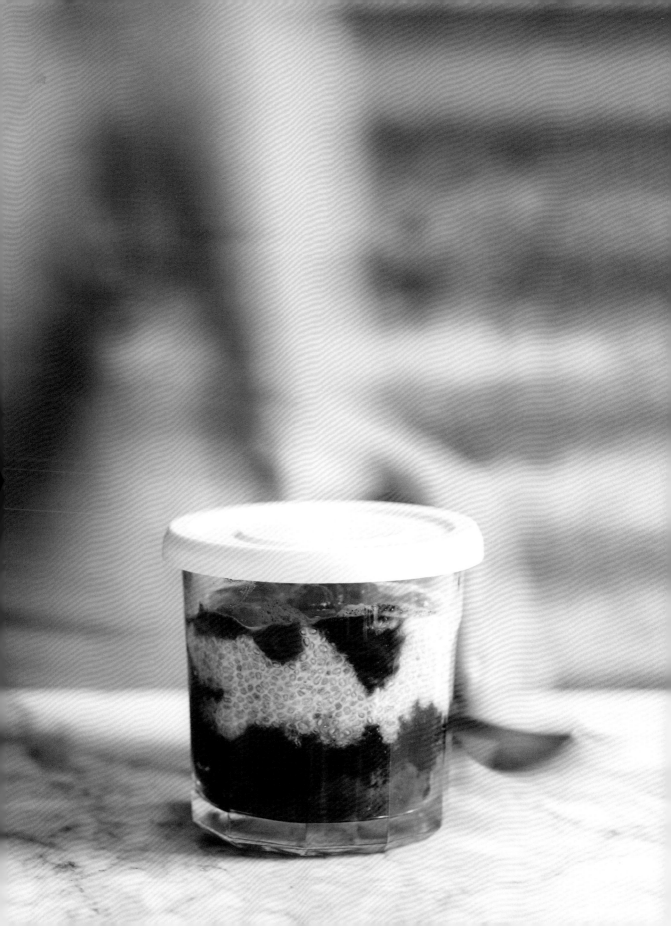

Really this is *the* easiest bread in the world to make and so quick. It takes 10 minutes to assemble and is ready in 1 hour. No yeast, no gluten, no wheat, this is a perfect one to make, slice up and then freeze so you always have nutritious bread at home. If you can't get teff, use ground almonds instead, or just gluten-free flour alone. The texture will not be the same, but the result is still delicious.

MAKES 1 LOAF

soda bread

Preheat the oven to 200°C/180°C fan/gas mark 6.

Flick some water into a heavy-duty casserole dish (about 21cm in diameter) and sprinkle in some gluten-free flour so that the sides and base of the pan are lightly coated. This will help to prevent the bread from sticking. Place the pan in the oven to heat up while you prepare the bread. By baking the bread in a pan like this, you will be sure to get a really delicious, crunchy crust.

Combine the almond (or other plant-based milk) with the apple cider vinegar in a jug. This is how you make a dairy-free 'buttermilk'. Leave to sit while you prepare the other ingredients.

In a bowl, combine the remaining ingredients and mix thoroughly. Make a well in the centre and then pour in the almond milk mixture. Use your hands to stir the mixture together until it forms a nice dough. Knead on a lightly floured surface for a minute or two. You want the dough to be as smooth as possible so that the bread does not crack when baked. Shape the dough into a circle roughly the same diameter as the pan.

Place the dough in the hot pan and sprinkle the top with a little extra gluten-free flour. Bake in the oven with the lid on for 55–60 minutes. The bread is ready if it sounds hollow inside when you tap it. Leave it to cool on a wire rack.

360ml almond or other plant milk (bought or see page 52)

1½ tbsp apple cider vinegar

2 tsp coconut palm sugar or syrup

225g gluten-free plain flour, plus extra for sprinkling

225g teff flour

2 tsp bicarbonate of soda

1 tsp baking powder

1 tbsp xanthan gum

½ tsp Himalayan pink salt

*

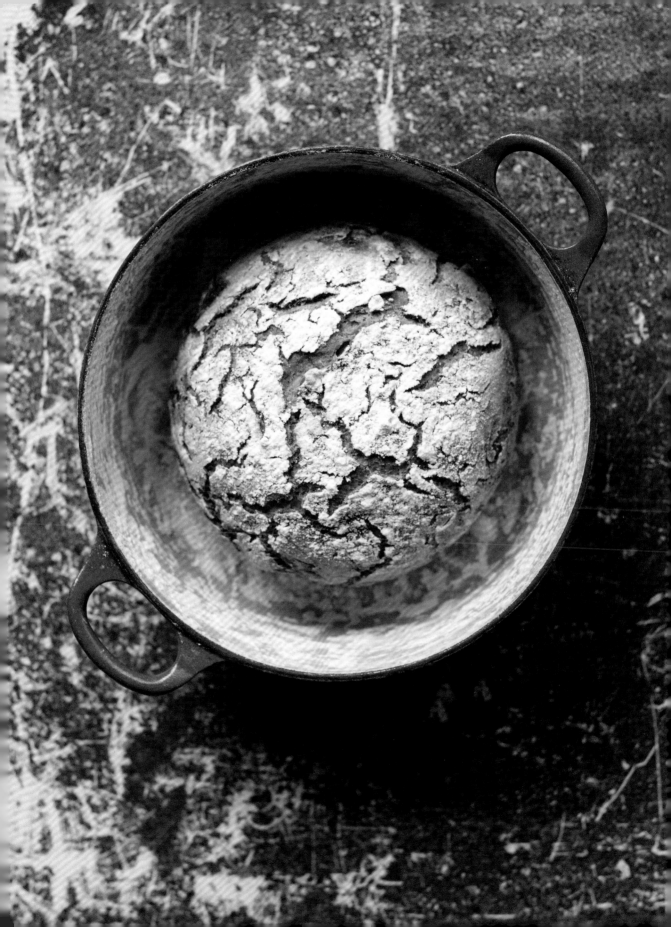

This is one of those recipes that I have not eaten since I was a child and now I have created a healthier version! It works best with a soft, gluten-free white bread as it will taste just like the real deal. However, if you can't find such a loaf, you can use the Soda bread on page 46 and leave to soak for longer as it is just as delicious.

SERVES 2

french blueberry toast

Beat together the egg, almond milk, vanilla and coconut palm sugar, if using, in a large mixing bowl. Dip the slices of bread in so they soak it all up (if you use soda bread, it won't soak up as much).

Heat the coconut oil in a frying pan, add the slices of eggy bread and place the blueberries along one side.

Leave to cook for 1 minute or until golden brown, then flip and cook the other side for another minute.

Serve with the warmed bursting blueberries over the top.

1 egg
60ml almond milk (bought or see page 52)
¼ tsp vanilla extract
1 tbsp coconut palm sugar, to make it sweeter (optional)
4 slices gluten-free bread or Soda bread (see page 46)
1 tbsp coconut oil
50g frozen or fresh blueberries

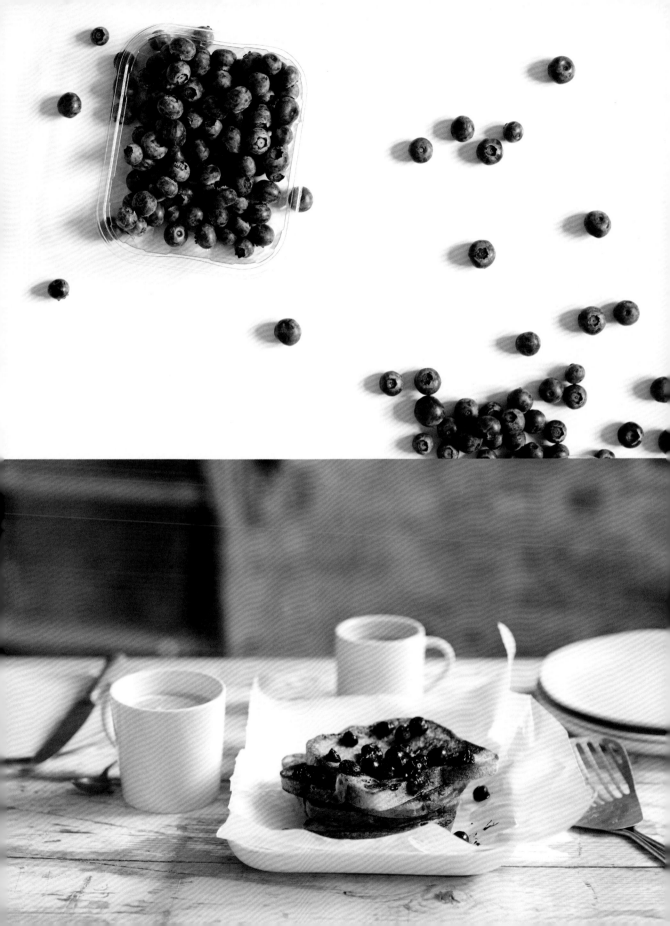

Sometimes I come down for a quick breakfast to find the granola jar empty, and it was during one of those moments that I created this very quick stove-top granola in 5 minutes. It's a lifesaver and packed with energy from the nuts and seeds. I love it with yoghurt or a splash of almond milk – the cacao makes the milk go all chocolaty, so what's not to love?

MAKES 320G TO FILL A SMALL KILNER JAR (6-8 PORTIONS)

cacao granola

Melt 1 tablespoon of the coconut oil in a heavy-bottomed saucepan (use your largest pan as the granola will crisp up more quickly).

Combine the remaining ingredients in a bowl and stir until incorporated.

Put half of the granola mixture into the saucepan and toast for 1–2 minutes until the nuts are nice and toasty and you start to smell that chocolaty, nut aroma.

Beware – once the colour starts to turn, the mixture can burn quite quickly, so keep an eye on it. Once it is nice and golden, transfer straight away to a baking tray to cool (this is quite an important step as the pan will be really hot and the mixture will keep cooking and burn if you leave it in there).

Toast the remaining half of the mixture with the remaining coconut oil and leave to cool and crisp up with the other half.

2 tbsp coconut oil
100g quinoa flakes
100g whole buckwheat groats
50g pecans, roughly chopped
50g whole almonds
1 tbsp raw cacao powder
1 tsp vanilla extract
4 tbsp agave or coconut
    blossom syrup
a generous pinch of
    Himalayan pink salt
some chopped dates or dried
    fruit for more sweetness
    (optional)

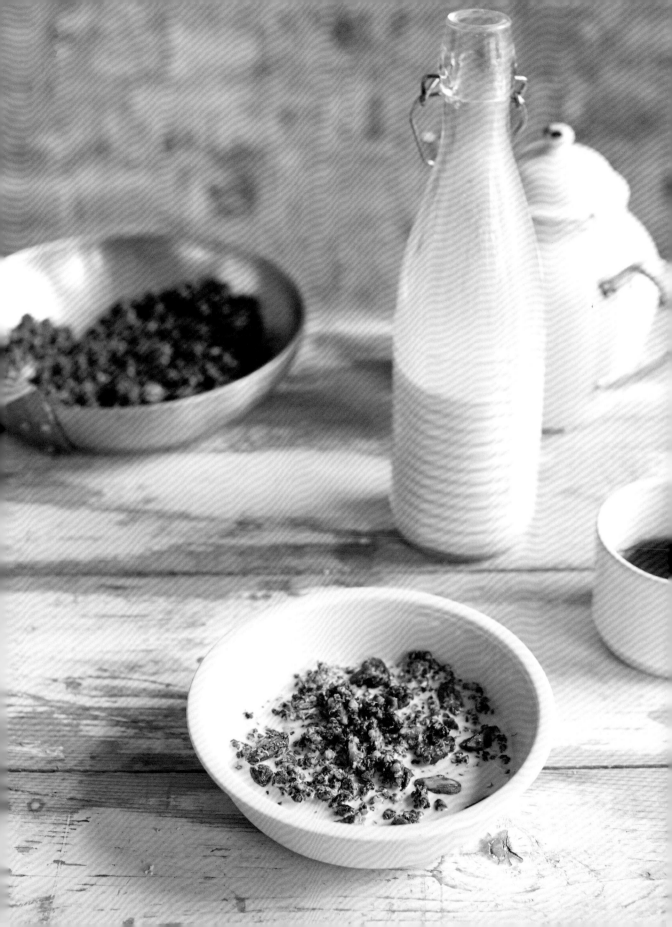

Making your own almond milk is so satisfying, and when you have done it once, you won't turn back. You can thin it out as much as you want – just add more water – but I love it quite thick and creamy. Add it to ice-creams (Manuka pollen maca ice-cream on page 218) and use the pulp for sweet treats (the Almond pulp chewy bites on page 186). This is a perfect recipe to have up your sleeve because I love the fact that if I have been away and have nothing in my fridge, I can soak some almonds overnight when I get home and have fresh milk in the morning for a bowl of porridge.

MAKES 750ML MILK

almond milk

Start by soaking the almonds – they need to be completely covered with cold water. Let them sit for at least 30 minutes before draining and transferring to a blender. Add 1 litre water to the blender and blitz until as smooth as possible.

Strain the mixture through a muslin bag over a large bowl. You will need to squeeze the bag to get out as much of the milk as possible. Loosen with more water if necessary to make the thickness you like. Transfer it from the bowl into a screwtop jar and keep in the fridge.

400g whole almonds
1 litre cold water

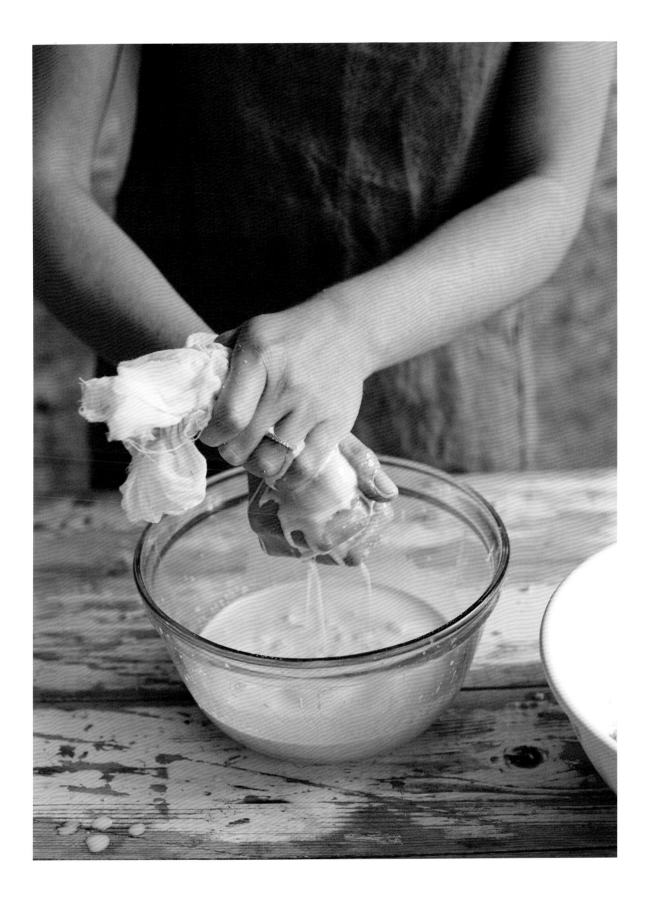

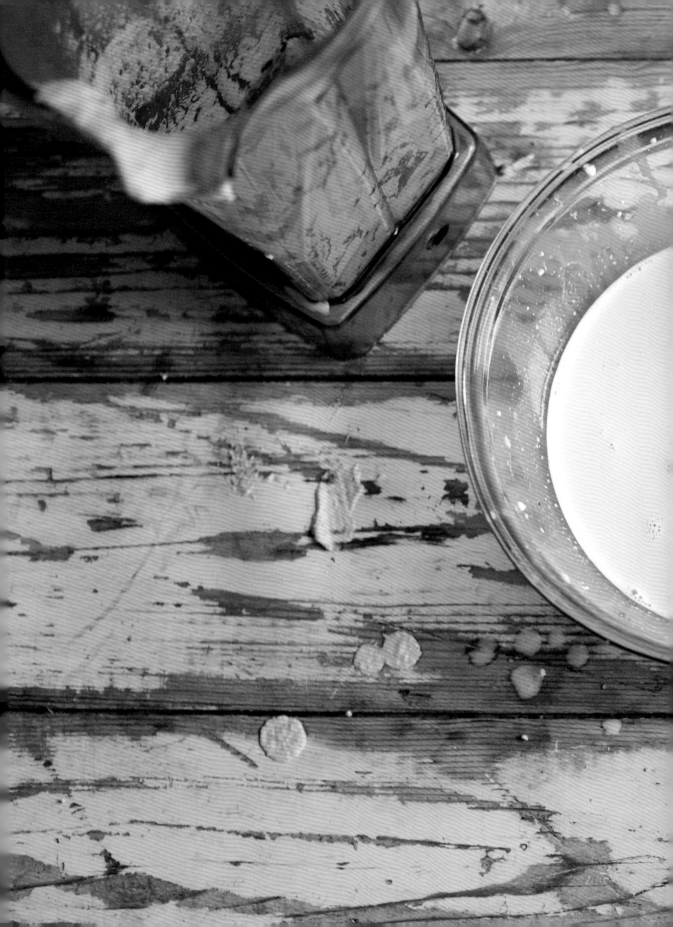

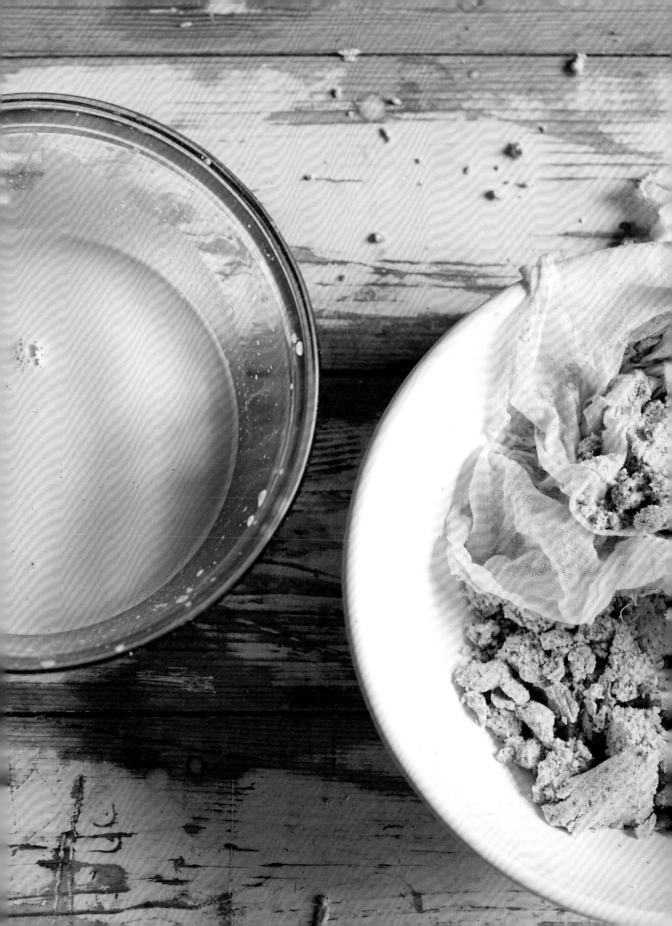

If you have ever made jam, you will know that it can take quite a
bit of work to get that jar of perfectly set fruit – with a ton of
sugar added in there too. This recipe could not be further from that.
It is so simple to make and there's no sugar required. I use frozen
blueberries, but fresh would work just as well. Spread the
jam on home-made Soda bread (see page 46) or pancakes
for one of the all-time best breakfasts.

MAKES 160G JAM

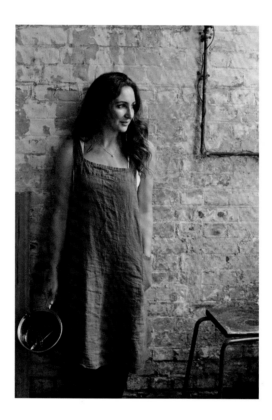

blueberry jam

Put the blueberries, agave and lemon zest into a pan and bring
to a gentle boil. Simmer for a further 10–12 minutes until the
juice has reduced and you have a nice thick mixture.

Store in a clean jar in the fridge for up to a week, or freeze and
defrost as needed.

250g blueberries (frozen or
fresh)
2 tsp agave syrup
zest of ¼ lemon

*

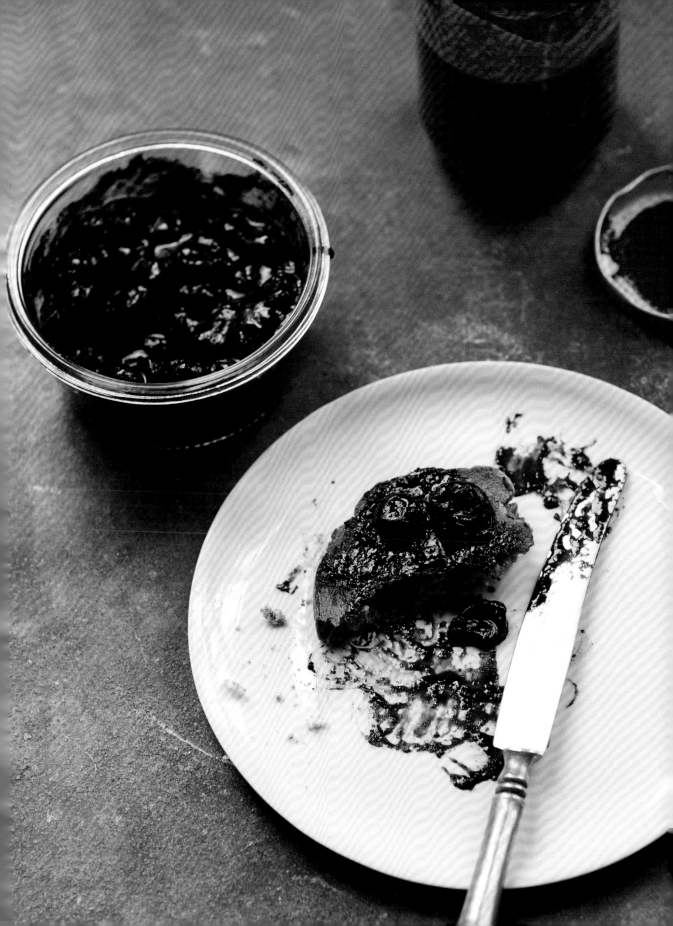

I love crumpets, and while I was developing the recipe
for my Tacos (see page 98), I put a little too much batter into
the pan and it came out thick and the texture of a
crumpet. That made me think I could adapt the recipe to
create a crumpet, and the end result is delicious. It reminds
me of coming back from a cold, wet walk and having
Marmite on crumpets with a big cup of tea!

MAKES 6 CRUMPETS

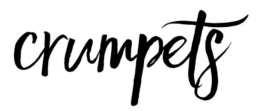

Heat the rice milk and 175ml water in a pan until it is a tepid
temperature. Take off the heat and add the sugar and dried
yeast. Mix, cover with a cloth and leave in a warm place for 10
minutes until it starts to froth up.

Combine the gluten-free flour, salt and baking powder in a
bowl. Make a well in the flour, pour in the frothy liquid and beat
together until it forms a thick batter.

Heat the coconut oil in a non-stick frying pan. Meanwhile,
grease the inside of an egg ring (silicone will work best) and
place in the pan (if you have more than one ring, you can cook
a few crumpets at a time). If you don't have an egg ring, you
can make your own with doubled strip of foil shaped to the
same size. It will be harder to get the foil off, so you will need
to cut it: just be careful as it will be very hot!

Spoon about 3 heaped tablespoons of batter into the ring and
leave to cook on a medium heat. When bubbles start to appear
and it looks like the batter is solid, which will take about 4–5
minutes, slowly ease off the ring, leaving the crumpet in the
pan. Flip it over to cook on the other side until golden. Repeat
with the remaining batter.

Serve the crumpets with some coconut oil and wonderful jam
or the Blueberry or Rhubarb Compote (see pages 44 or 197).

175ml rice milk
1 tbsp coconut sugar
½ tsp dried yeast
225g gluten-free plain flour
½ tsp Himalayan pink salt
1½ tsp baking powder
1 tbsp coconut oil, for
    cooking

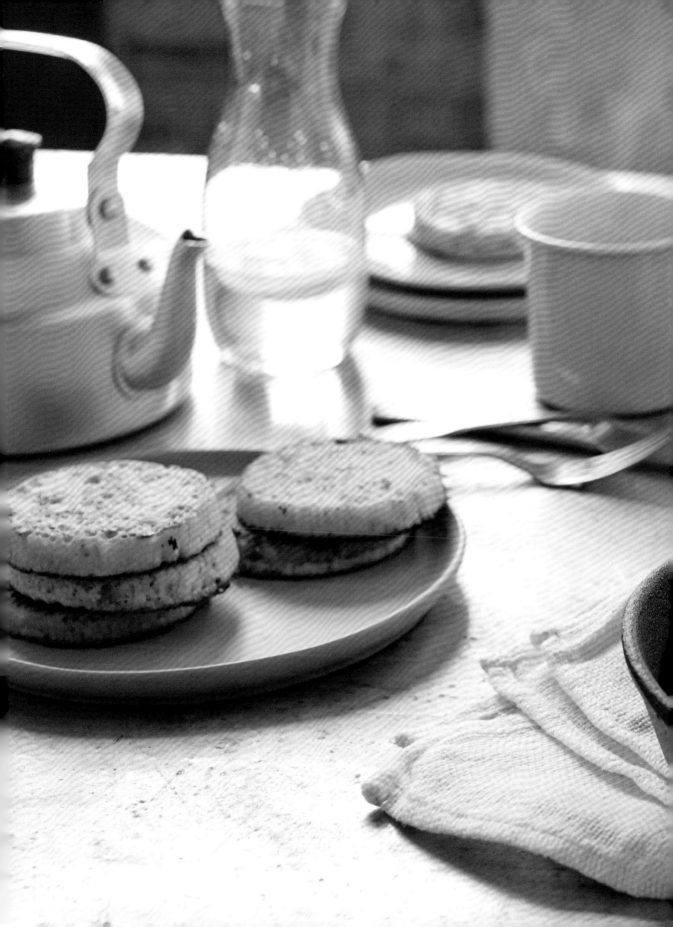

Turmeric really is such a fantastic ingredient and the huge range
of things that it does for our bodies is incredible. It is also a natural
stimulant and helps to boost your immune system.

SERVES 1

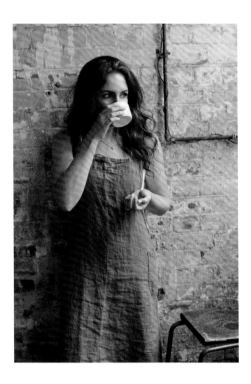

turmeric
tea

Put the fennel seeds into a pan with 400ml water and simmer
for 1 minute. Add the remaining ingredients, bring to the boil
and simmer for a further minute. Strain and drink piping hot.

½ tsp fennel seeds
2cm piece of fresh turmeric,
   finely chopped
2 slices of lemon
3 slices of root ginger

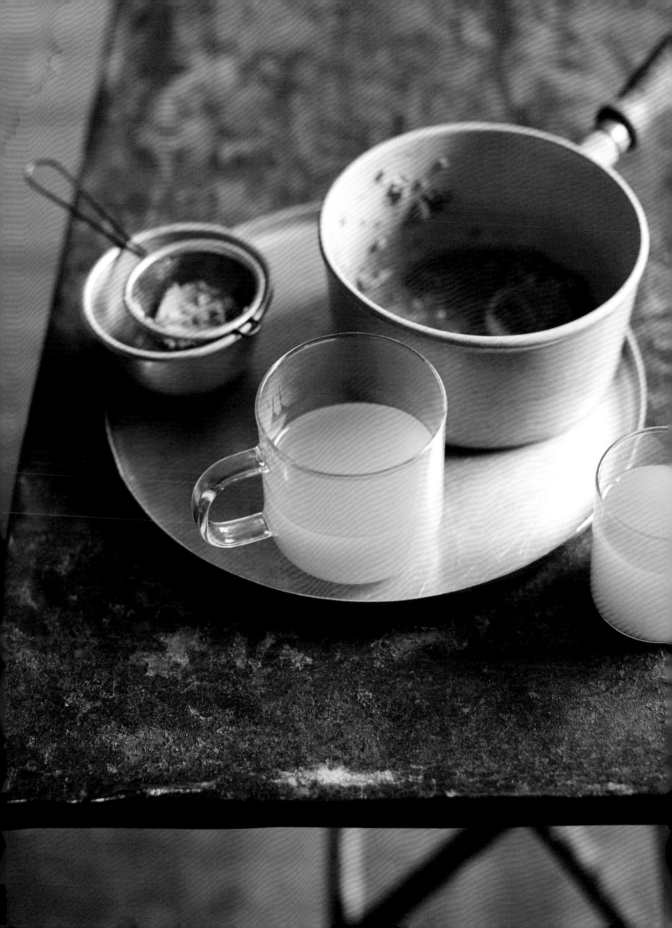

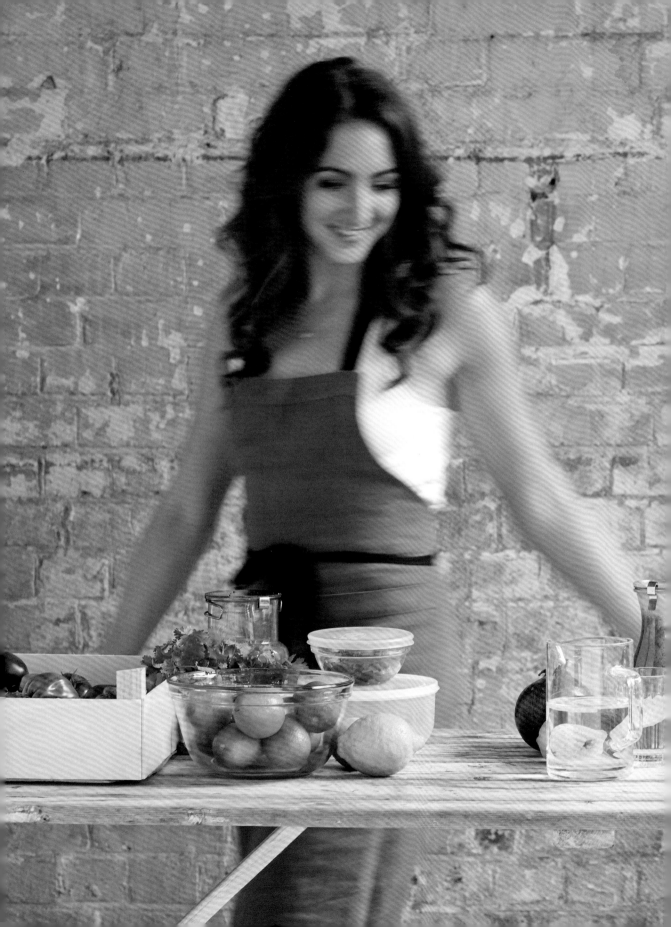

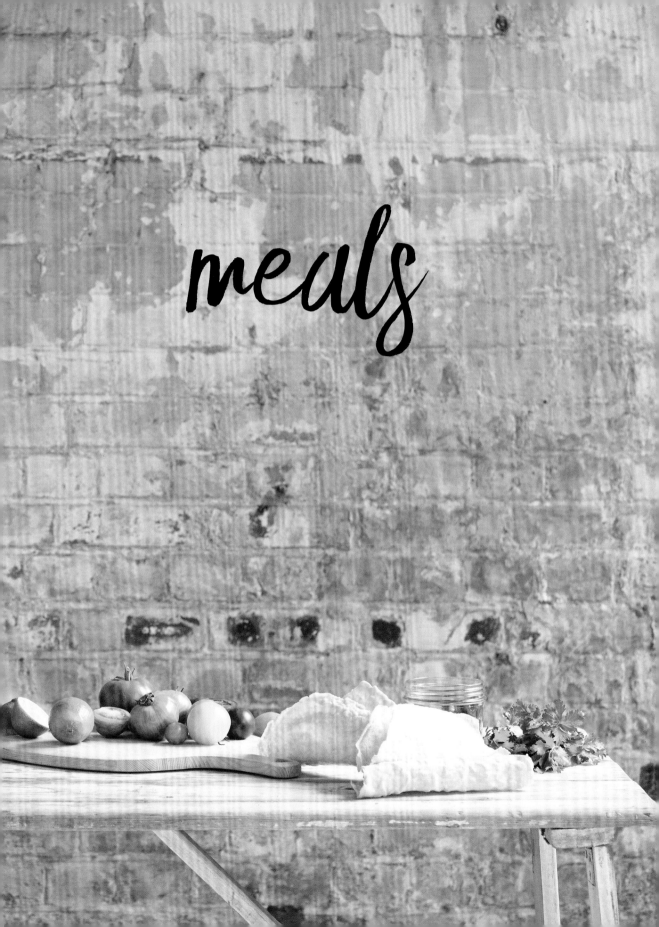

meals

Travelling is a huge part of the way I get my inspiration.
As I have always loved Asian food, it was never going to be
long before I wanted to re-create this traditional soup –
known as *tom kha* in Thailand. It is full of flavour and very
quick to make. The coconut gives it such a thick and creamy
texture, making it feel naughty, but you know it's so
good for you with all those essential fats.

MAKES 1 LARGE OR 2 SMALL PORTIONS

thai coconut soup

In a saucepan, sauté the garlic, lemongrass and ginger in the coconut oil for 2 minutes, stirring constantly.

Add the coconut milk, chilli slices, brown rice vinegar and lime zest and simmer for 4 minutes to combine all the flavours.

Add 200ml water, half the lime juice and the baby tomatoes. Leave to cook on a medium heat for 4 minutes – you want the tomatoes to burst their skin.

Add the mushrooms and, after a minute, add the bok choy and cook for another minute. Season with the salt, sprinkle over the coriander and remaining lime juice to taste, and serve piping hot.

2 cloves garlic, grated
1 lemongrass stalk, sliced
5cm piece of root ginger, grated
1 tsp coconut oil
400ml coconut milk
2–3cm piece of chilli, sliced
¼ tsp brown rice vinegar
zest and juice of 1 lime
80g baby tomatoes
60g mushrooms
100g bok choy, leaves separated
a pinch of Himalayan pink salt
5g fresh coriander

Add rice noodles for a more filling meal.

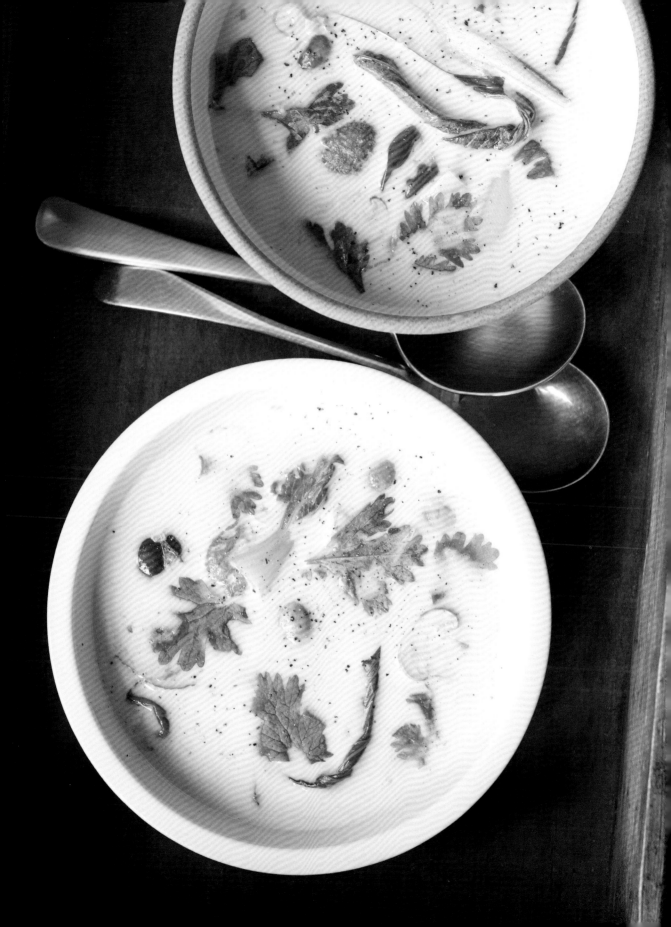

This aromatic, warming soup reminds me of winter and Sundays at home when I was little. The rosemary and garlic have such a wonderfully fragrant smell. Butternut is a very alkaline ingredient and, coupled with fennel, can help to reduce bloating and water retention. You can make this soup in bulk and freeze in portion bags so that you always have something nourishing and healthy to come home to even if you don't have anything in your fridge.

SERVES 2

butternut, fennel AND ginger soup

Sauté the red onion, garlic, ginger and cumin seeds in the sunflower oil for 2 minutes. Add the sprig of rosemary, keeping it whole so that it's easy to remove later.

Make the stock by combining the vegetable bouillon powder with 500ml hot water.

Add 4 tablespoons of your stock to the pan and leave to simmer on a medium to low heat for 2 minutes. Then add another 4 tablespoons of stock and leave for a further 2 minutes. This technique of 'layering' helps to make a wonderful flavour.

Leave to simmer for another 2 minutes, then add the butternut squash and the rest of the stock. Leave on a medium heat for 10 minutes before adding the chopped fennel and another 200ml hot water.

Simmer for another 10-12 minutes until both the fennel and butternut are nice and soft.

Take the rosemary stalk out and then add a pinch of salt to taste. Transfer the contents of the pan to a blender and whizz until velvety smooth before serving.

1 small red onion, diced
1 clove garlic, finely chopped
5cm piece of root ginger, sliced
1 tsp cumin seeds
1 tbsp sunflower or coconut oil
1 sprig of rosemary, plus extra to garnish
1 tbsp vegetable bouillon powder
450g butternut squash, cut into 2cm cubes
160g fennel, cut into 2cm cubes
a pinch of Himalayan pink salt
rosemary leaves and cumin seeds, to garnish (optional)

You can garnish this soup with some crispy rosemary and cumin seeds, baked for 5-6 minutes in an oven preheated to 180°C/160°C fan/gas mark 4.

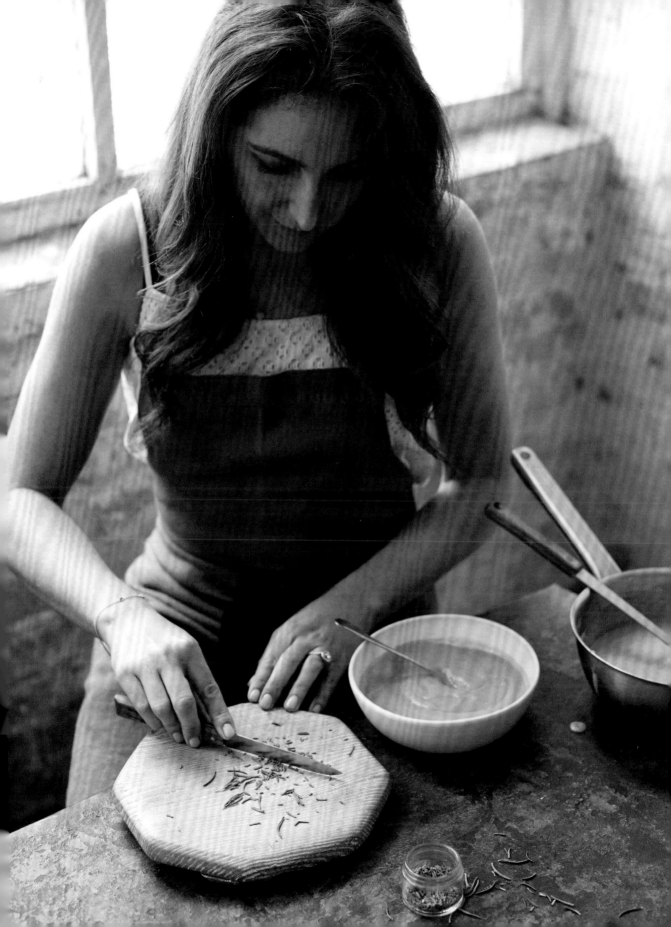

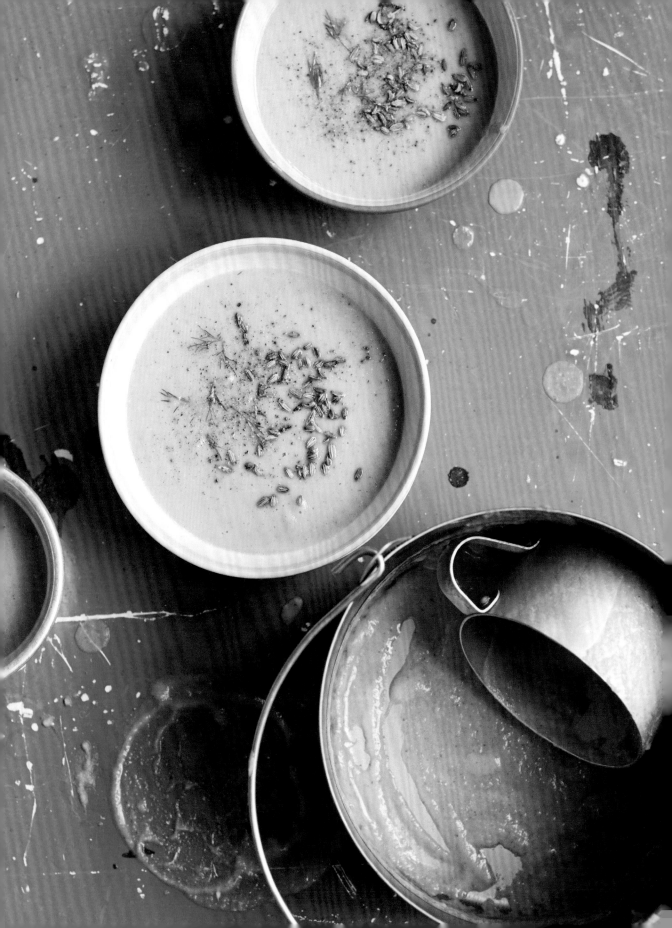

If you want nourishment in a bowl in 10 minutes, then this warming and velvety soup is for you. Vibrantly green and full of flavour, it is one of my go-to easy suppers that really fills you up. If you are cooking for one, don't forget to freeze the other portion and you can go back to it when you have no food in the fridge!

SERVES 2

broccoli soup

1 clove garlic, roughly chopped
110g leeks, chopped into pieces
½ tsp fennel seeds, plus extra to garnish
1 tbsp coconut oil
500ml boiling water
1 tsp bouillon powder
270g broccoli, cut into florets
5g dill
a pinch of Himalayan pink salt

Sauté the garlic, leeks and fennel seeds in the coconut oil for 2 minutes. Add the boiling water and bouillon powder, bring to the boil and simmer for 2 minutes.

Add the broccoli and cook for 4 minutes until soft.

Take off the heat, add the dill, pour into a blender and whizz until smooth. Add salt to taste and blend once more.

Garnish with fennel seeds.

You can swap the broccoli for any soft green vegetable. Try beans, peas, kale, spinach or asparagus for different tastes.

When spring vegetables come into season, we still have some chilly evenings in the UK, so I love a delicious chunky soup to warm me up. If you don't want to make your own pesto, you can use shop-bought, but it really is quick and simple to make. It also means you can freeze it and keep for a rainy day to add to pasta!

SERVES 2

spring minestrone soup

Sauté the red onion and garlic in the sunflower oil for 1 minute. Add the pesto and 60ml of the water and leave to simmer for 2 minutes.

Add the rest of the boiling water and the vegetable bouillon powder and bring to a simmer. Add the sprouting broccoli, courgettes and tomatoes and leave to cook for 2 minutes. Add the frozen peas, wild garlic/spinach, lemon juice, chives and salt and pepper. Stir through and simmer for a further minute, then remove from the heat.

Serve with a garnish of additional chives over the top.

½ red onion, finely chopped

1 clove garlic, finely chopped

1 tsp sunflower oil

70g pesto (use the frozen cubes of Perfect pesto on page 181)

600ml boiling water

1 tbsp vegetable bouillon powder

80g sprouting broccoli, chopped into 5 × 5mm strips

100g courgettes, cut into 1cm cubes

100g cherry tomatoes, halved

90g frozen peas

50g wild garlic (or spinach leaves)

juice of ½ lemon

5g chives, chopped, plus extra to garnish

Himalayan pink salt and freshly ground black pepper

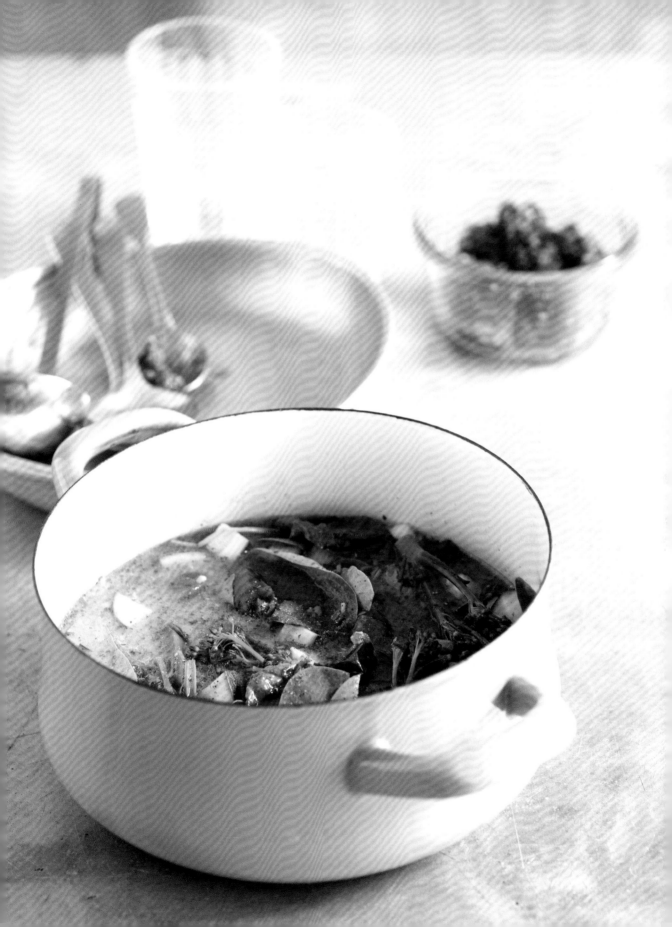

This is honestly one of the most warming and satisfying
soups ever. There is something about the rich caramelised flavours that
just sort you out after a long day. This recipe does require fairly slow
cooking, but it is the type you can leave simmering while you buzz about
doing other things. It also happens to be incredibly good value, so if you
are cooking on a budget, then this is definitely a recipe for you.

SERVES 2

french onion soup

Peel and slice the onions. This step might make you cry a bit, so a little tip is to run the peeled onions under cold water before slicing them. Or wear some goggles!

Melt the vegan butter in a large saucepan and then add the onions. Cover the pan and sweat the onions over a gentle heat for 7–8 minutes until the slices are nice and soft.

Remove the lid and continue to cook the onion slices so that they develop a really beautiful caramelised colour. This stage should take about 35–40 minutes. Be careful to stir the onions every now and then as you do not want them to burn – but at the same time, hold your nerve as you want them to go a lovely dark brown for maximum flavour.

Once nice and brown, stir through the mirin, vegetable bouillon powder and 600ml boiling water. Season to taste with salt and pepper.

Turn on your grill to a medium-high heat.

Ladle the soup into bowls and place a slice of gluten-free toast onto each. Sprinkle the cheese over it and grill for 10–12 minutes or until beautifully golden brown. Serve piping hot.

870g onions
3 tbsp soft vegan butter
1 tsp mirin
2 tsp vegetable bouillon powder
600ml boiling water
Himalayan pink salt and freshly ground black pepper

for the topping:
2 slices gluten-free bread, toasted
70g soft goats' or feta cheese, crumbled

>>●

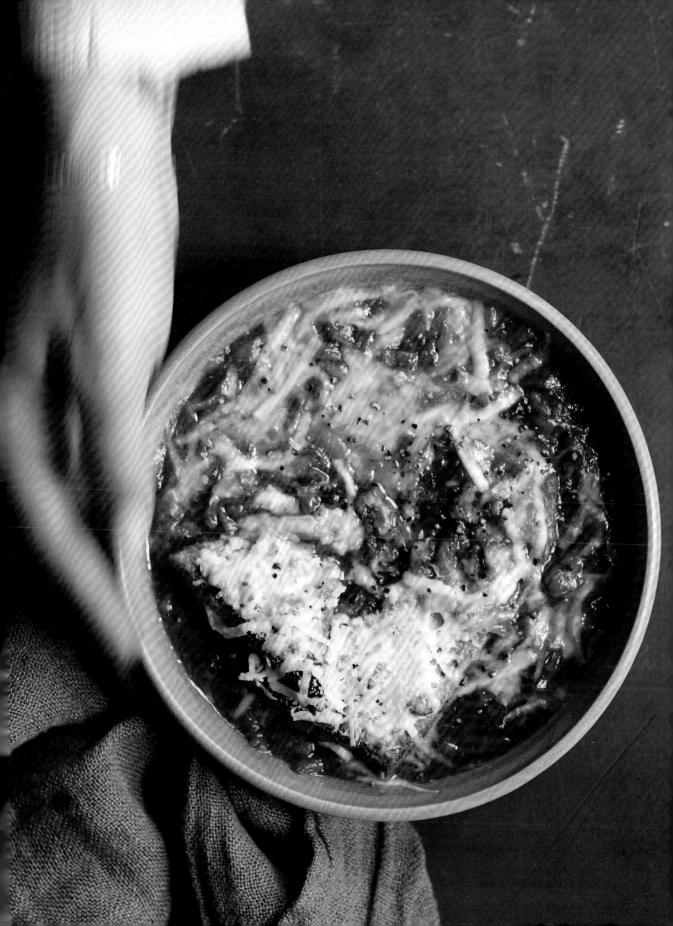

Sometimes all I fancy is a warming broth that I know is good
for me with a little substance that is not going to bloat me.
I love cooking with miso because it's fermented and great for
the gut, but it also tastes delicious.

SERVES 2

cucumber noodle asparagus broth

To soft-boil the eggs, cook them in a pan of boiling water for 6 minutes. Run under cold water and peel the shells off.

Sauté the garlic, ginger and coriander in the coconut oil in a medium saucepan for 1 minute. Add 125ml water and cook for another 2 minutes. Add the brown rice miso, lime zest and the 400ml boiling water, bring to the boil, then simmer for 3 minutes.

Add the lime juice, apple cider vinegar and asparagus and cook for 1 minute. Just before serving, put the spiralised cucumber noodles into the broth with the spring onion and mint. Cut the egg in half, place on the top and garnish with a little cracked pepper.

2 eggs

1 clove garlic, finely chopped

2.5cm piece of root ginger, sliced

¼ tsp ground coriander

1 tsp coconut oil

1 tbsp brown rice miso

zest of 1 lime

400ml boiling water

juice of ½ lime

¼ tsp apple cider vinegar

100g asparagus, sliced lengthways then chopped in half

190g cucumber, spiralised

1 large or 2 small spring onions, thinly sliced

5g mint leaves

freshly ground black pepper

I use a spiraliser here as it makes brilliant long noodles out of vegetables like courgettes, cucumbers and carrots. If you don't have one, you could use a peeler to make long strips and then slice these into noodles.

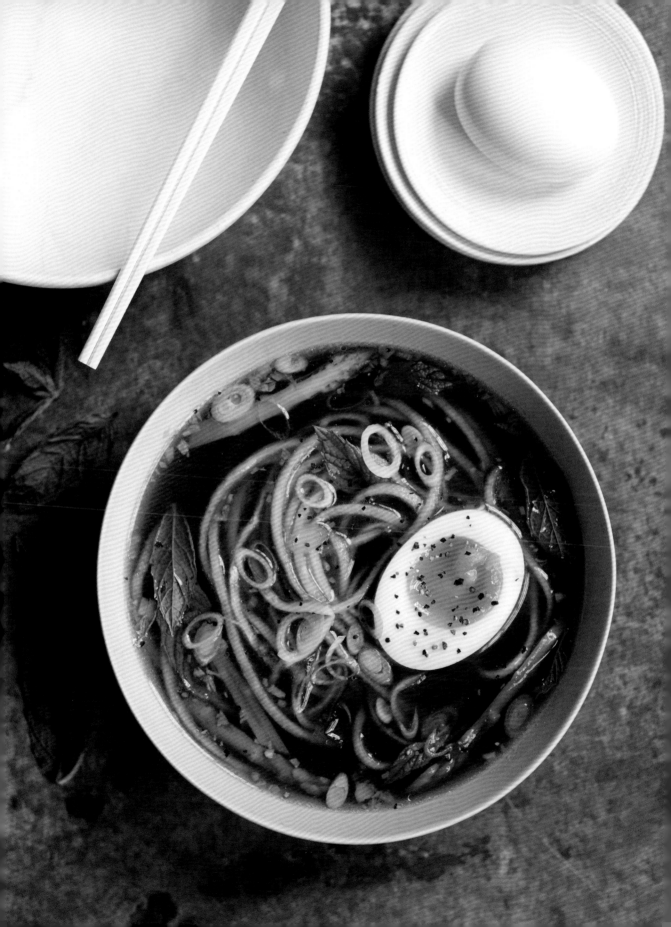

This is a delicious, healthy alternative to a traditional avocado mousse. The agar flakes are used to set the mousse like gelatine would, but they are made from seaweed, are great for digestion and really alkaline. You can also use them for making a healthy vegan jelly. This mousse is a great standby in your fridge – perfect to add to a salad or sandwich to take to work.

SERVES 2

avocado mousse

In a pan, mix together the bouillon powder and the boiling water until dissolved. Scatter the agar flakes over the top of the stock, put onto the heat and bring to the boil. Do not stir until the mixture has come to the boil and you have then turned the heat off.

In a blender, mix together the avocado, lemon juice, grated garlic, pink salt and coconut cream until smooth. Mix in the stock and blend again.

Stir in the chopped dill and pour into two ramekins or glasses. Place in the fridge to set for 2 hours.

Serve with toasted gluten-free bread.

1 tbsp vegetable bouillon powder
75ml boiling water
1 tbsp agar flakes
1 avocado, peeled and stone removed
juice of ½ lemon
1 clove garlic, finely grated
a pinch of Himalayan pink salt
75ml coconut cream (or the creamy top from a can of coconut milk)
5g dill, roughly chopped

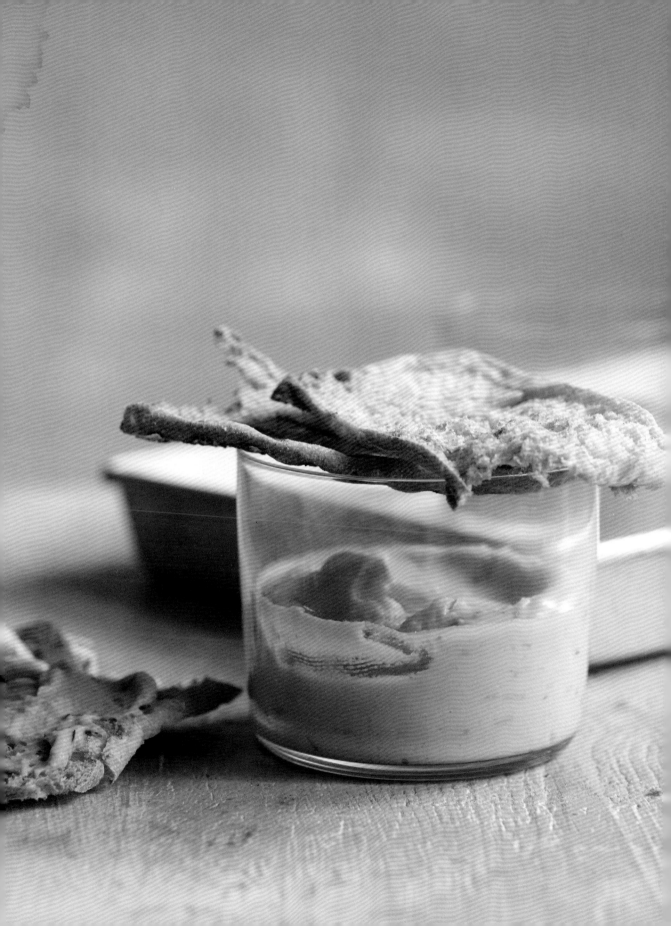

I love using spices in all my dishes, especially in rice
dishes as I am hugely influenced by Middle Eastern cooking.
This salad is so simple and really punches with flavour.

SERVES 2-4

middle eastern potato salad

First make the dressing by mixing the cinnamon, cumin, pinch of salt and yoghurt together.

Arrange the cooled sweet potato on a platter, pour the dressing over it and sprinkle with the chopped parsley. Serve with a salad or as a side dish, garnished with the pomegranate seeds if you like.

350g roasted sweet potato, cooled (550g raw sweet potato, quartered lengthways) (see page 12)
10g parsley, chopped
pomegranate seeds, to garnish (optional)

for the dressing:
½ tsp ground cinnamon
1 tsp ground cumin
¼ tsp Himalayan pink salt
250g goats' or sheeps' milk yoghurt

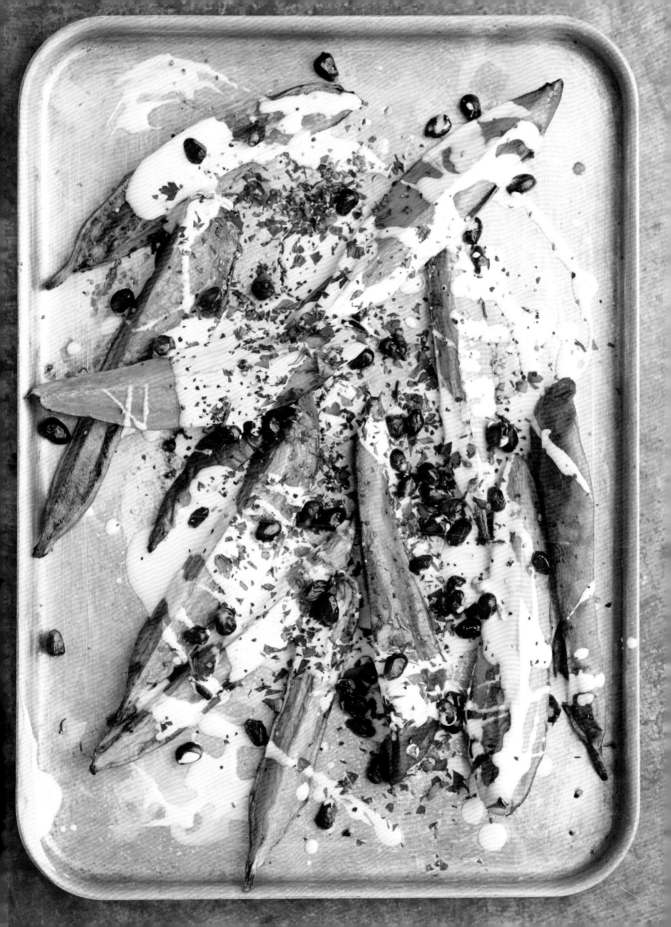

Teff is an amazing grain – one of my favourites. It is used a lot in
African cooking, so I thought an African Teff Stew would be
just the thing. Okra is another traditional African vegetable and is
something I should really cook with more as it is so delicious.

SERVES 2

african teff stew

Put the red onion, garlic, turmeric, cumin, ginger and sunflower
oil in a pan and sauté over a medium heat for about a minute.
Add 60ml water and once this has reduced down, add
another 60ml water, chilli and the tomatoes and cook for a
further 2 minutes.

Next add the butternut squash, 700ml water and the vegetable
bouillon powder and simmer for 5 minutes before adding the
teff and continuing to cook for a further 15 minutes.

When the butternut is soft, season the stew with salt and
pepper and stir through the okra and kale. Cook for a further
4–5 minutes until the okra is just soft.

Serve the stew as it is or with a little yogurt on top.

1 red onion, diced

1 clove garlic, roughly
    chopped

½ tsp ground turmeric or
    2.5cm piece of fresh
    turmeric, grated

1 tsp ground cumin

3cm piece of root ginger,
    finely chopped

1 tbsp sunflower oil

250g tomatoes, roughly
    chopped

½ red chilli, cut in half
    lengthways

300g butternut squash, cut
    into 2cm cubes

2 tsp vegetable bouillon
    powder

80g whole teff grain

a pinch of Himalayan pink salt

freshly ground black pepper

70g okra, chopped into 4cm
    pieces (if you can't find
    okra, use courgettes)

50g kale, roughly chopped

yoghurt, to serve (optional)

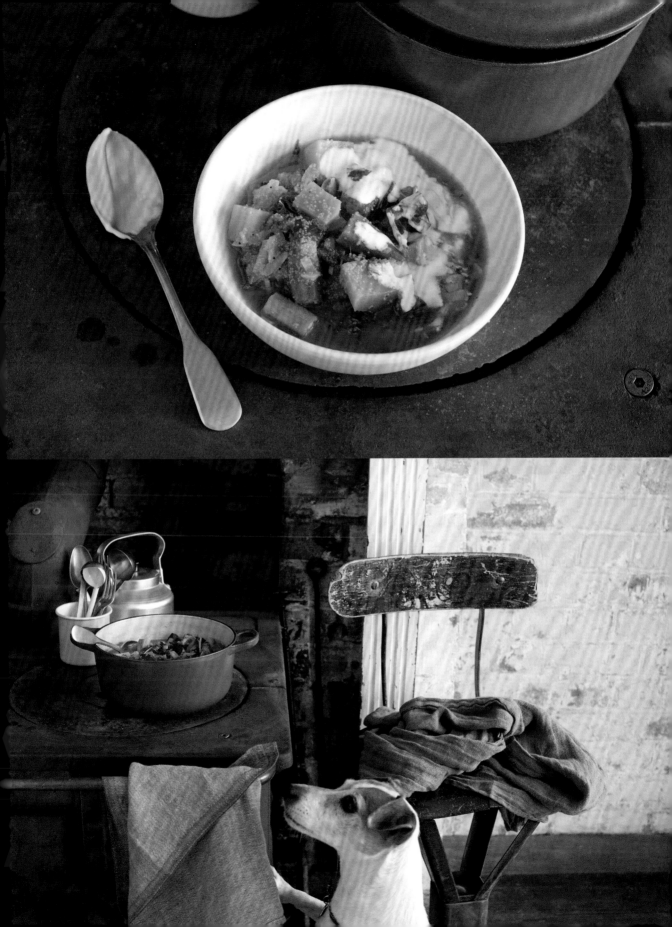

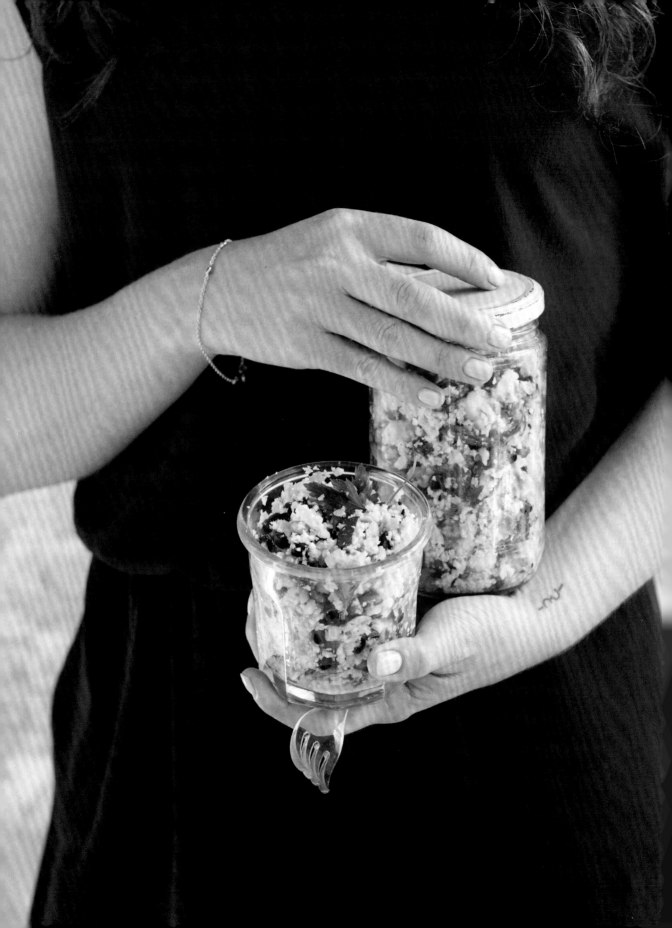

This is a great side dish to add to your main meal as a healthy alternative to heavy carbohydrates. I love it with grilled tofu or with my Blistered aubergine and courgette (see page 144). It is also delicious with some wild rocket mixed through. Double up the quantities and use half later in the week to make my Tagine and cauli couscous (see page 85).

SERVES 2-3

israeli cauli couscous

1 whole (670g) cauliflower
1 red onion, diced
1 clove garlic, grated
1 tbsp sunflower oil
1 courgette (roughly 200g),
    cut into 1cm cubes
1 tsp ground coriander
¼ tsp nigella seeds
400ml stock (made with 1
    tbsp vegetable bouillon
    powder)
80g dried apricots, sliced
1 tsp brown rice vinegar
60g almonds
35g parsley, roughly chopped
juice of ½ lemon
zest of 1 lemon
seeds from ½ pomegranate
Himalayan pink salt
freshly ground black pepper
¼ tsp ground cumin

Start by blitzing the cauliflower in a food processor until it resembles the texture of short-grain rice. Set aside.

Sauté the onion and garlic in the sunflower oil in a pan over a medium heat for 2 minutes. Add the courgette, ground coriander and nigella seeds and continue to sauté for a further 2 minutes.

Add 100ml of the stock to the pan along with the cauliflower rice and stir over the heat for 2 minutes.

Add the dried apricots, brown rice vinegar and remaining stock and cook for a further 4 minutes. Add the almonds to warm for a few seconds and let any more moisture be absorbed by the cauliflower.

Remove the pan from the heat and stir through the parsley, lemon juice and zest, pomegranate seeds and seasoning to taste. Sprinkle the top with the ground cumin and serve.

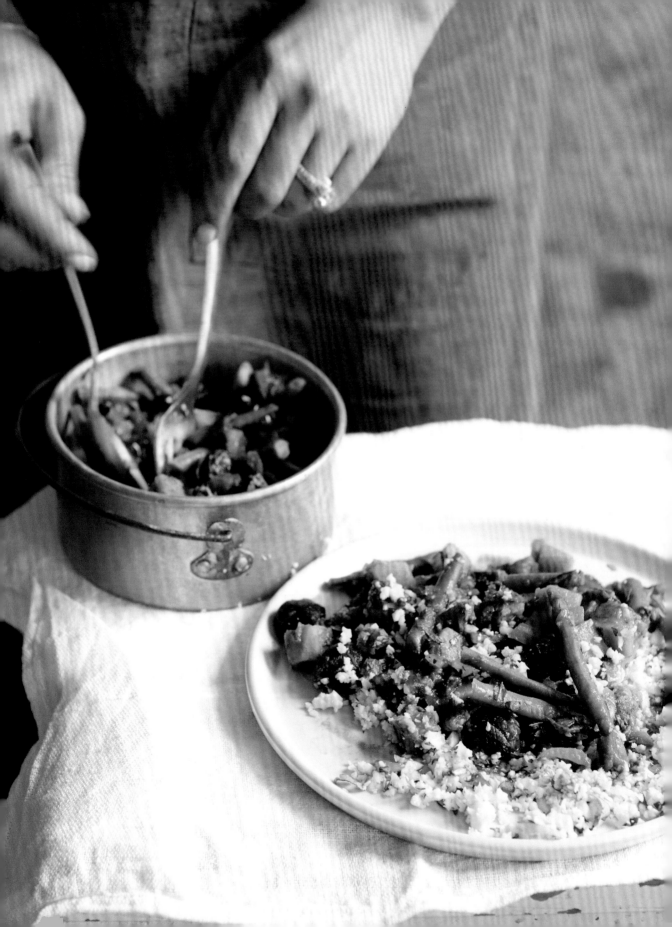

This perfectly warming tagine is a great quick-and-easy dish. You can play around with the ingredients, such as adding sweet potato or beetroot instead of the butternut squash. It takes about 20 minutes to make from scratch, but when you use roasted butternut squash from your prep night, it is ready in 10 minutes. This cauli couscous is a simpler version of my Israeli cauli couscous (see page 83). If you have cooked some extra of that recipe, you could use it here to make this dish even quicker to put together.

SERVES 2–3

tagine *and* cauli couscous

2 cloves garlic, grated

1 red onion, diced

1 tbsp sunflower oil

½ tsp ground cinnamon

½ tsp ground coriander

½ tsp ground cumin

460g vine tomatoes, chopped

150g roasted butternut
    squash (200g raw
    butternut squash, peeled
    and chopped into 1cm
    cubes) (see page 12)

100g green beans, topped and
    tailed

50g black olives

Himalayan pink salt

15g coriander, roughly
    chopped

for the cauli couscous:

360g cauliflower

1 tbsp sunflower oil

1 clove garlic, finely sliced

1 tsp cumin seeds

15g coriander, roughly
    chopped

10g mint, roughly chopped

a pinch of Himalayan pink salt

freshly ground black pepper

In a saucepan, sauté the grated garlic and the onion in the sunflower oil for 2 minutes. Add 60ml water and the cinnamon, ground coriander and cumin and heat for a further 2 minutes to cook out the spices.

Add the chopped tomatoes and coat in all the delicious spices. Add 125ml water and leave the pan to come up to a high temperature for 4 minutes until the water starts to be absorbed.

Add another 125ml water and the butternut squash, put the lid on and cook for 2 minutes.

Add the green beans with the black olives and season with salt. Stir and put the lid back on for another 2 minutes, then take off the heat and stir through the chopped coriander.

To make the cauli couscous, put the cauliflower in a food processor until it resembles the texture of short-grain rice. If you don't have a food processor, use a grater.

Put the sunflower oil in a frying pan and sauté the garlic and cumin seeds for 1 minute. Add the cauli couscous to the pan and mix in the coriander and mint. Season with salt and pepper. Leave to cook for 2 minutes, then take off heat.

Serve the cauli couscous with the tagine.

1+2 ❯

I had leftover quinoa and sweet potato in the fridge when I came home
one night and decided to see if I could throw them together to make
a risotto of sorts. It worked beautifully and is now one of my go-to dishes.
The best part about it is that a normal risotto can take 30–40 minutes
(even longer with brown rice) and requires lots of time spent stirring – while
this little number takes just 10 minutes! Add in the antioxidant power
of some fresh turmeric for added health benefits.

SERVES 2

ten-minute turmeric quinoa risotto

Put the onion, garlic, turmeric, fennel seeds and sunflower oil
into a wide-bottomed frying pan and sauté for 2 minutes until
soft. The wider the pan, the quicker the risotto will cook.

Add 250ml water and the vegetable bouillon powder and
simmer for a minute before adding the tomatoes. Cover and
continue to heat for a further 4 minutes until the tomatoes start
to break down.

Add the roasted sweet potato to the pan with a further
125ml water. Use the back of your spoon or spatula to break
down any larger bits of tomato or sweet potato – watch out
for splashes. You want to make sure that it's really smooth
and completely break down any lumps. Once it is a lovely
thick mixture, add a final 125ml water and the quinoa and s
tir through.

Add the salt and pepper and leave on the heat for a further
3 minutes or until you get a thick, risotto-like texture. Stir
through the grated cheese (or nutritional yeast), lemon zest
and juice and serve nice and hot.

½ white onion, diced

2 cloves garlic, finely sliced

5cm piece of fresh turmeric,
grated, or 1 tbsp ground
turmeric

½ tsp fennel seeds

1 tbsp sunflower oil

1 tbsp vegetable bouillon
powder

180g cherry tomatoes, cut
in half

170g roasted sweet potato
(250g raw sweet potato,
peeled and roughly
chopped) (see page 12)

190g precooked quinoa (100g
uncooked quinoa) (see
page 12)

a generous pinch of
Himalayan pink salt

a generous pinch of freshly
ground black pepper

30g hard goats' cheese or
pecorino, grated, or 2 tbsp
nutritional yeast

juice and zest of ½ lemon

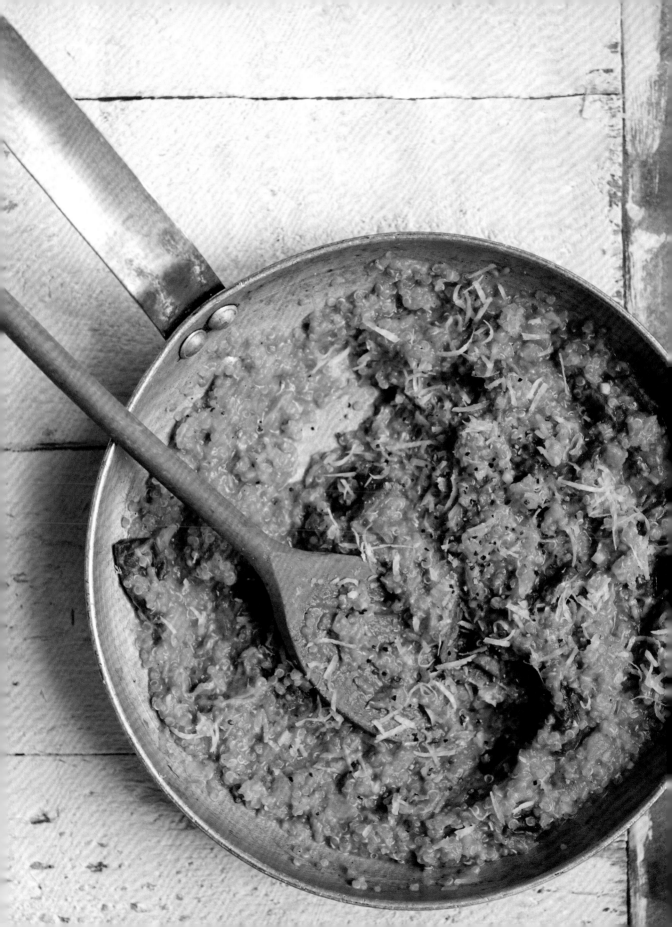

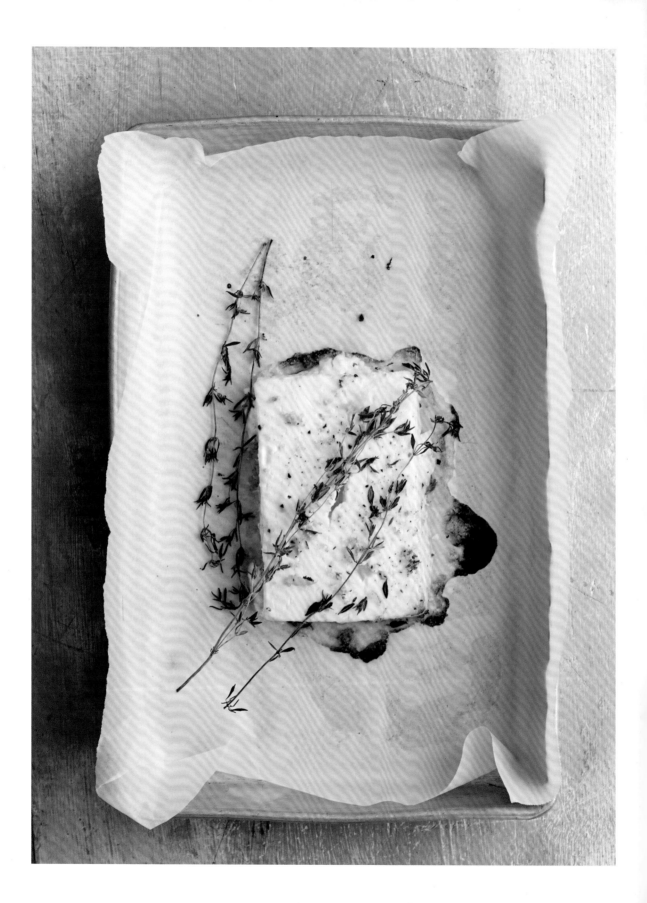

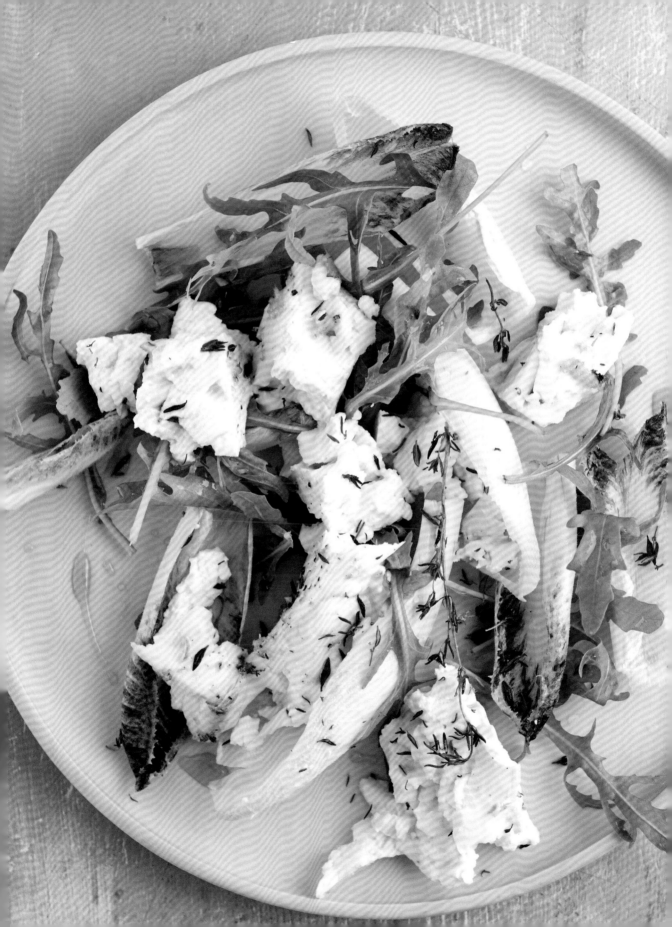

I have become slightly obsessed with baked feta and there
is a good reason! Not everyone likes the bitterness of chicory,
so you can just add more rocket or a different leaf to give it
that crunch with the softness of the warm feta.

SERVES 2

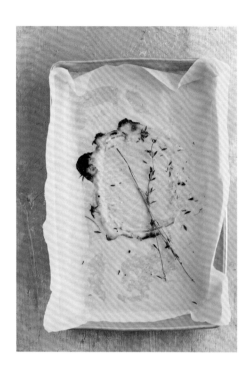

baked feta thyme salad

Preheat the oven to 170°C/150°C fan/gas mark 3.

Line a baking tray with greaseproof paper and place the whole
block of feta on it. Put the thyme on top with the lemon zest
and a pinch of pepper. Bake in the oven for 10 minutes.

Place the rocket and chicory on a plate, crumble the warm feta
over the top and drizzle with the sesame oil.

200g feta cheese
1 sprig of thyme
zest of 1 lemon
a pinch of freshly ground
   black pepper
70g rocket
70g red chicory
1 tsp sesame oil

This would be a great complement to any
Sunday roast or family lunch. It is zesty and punches above
its weight on flavour. You can turn this recipe into a
QUICK by using roasted cauliflower from your prep night
instead of the lemon-scented cauliflower below.

SERVES 2

roasted cauliflower *and* green bean sweet salad

500g cauliflower florets or
   350g roasted cauliflower
   florets (see page 12)
zest of 1 lemon and juice of
   ½ lemon
2 tsp walnut or sunflower oil
1 tsp sunflower oil
Himalayan pink salt
150g green beans, topped and
   tailed
10g dill, chopped
35g shelled pistachios
1 tsp pomegranate molasses
1 tbsp olive oil
a pinch of freshly ground
   black pepper
a pinch of sumac (optional)

Preheat the oven to 180°C/160°C fan/gas mark 4.

If using raw cauliflower florets put them on a baking tray and cover with the lemon zest, walnut and sunflower oils and a pinch of salt. Roast in the oven for 40 minutes until soft and slightly browning on the edges.

Blanch the green beans for 3 minutes in salted boiling water and drain.

Put the cauliflower, green beans, dill, pistachios, pomegranate molasses, olive oil, lemon juice, pepper, sumac (if using) and another pinch of salt into a dish and mix together.

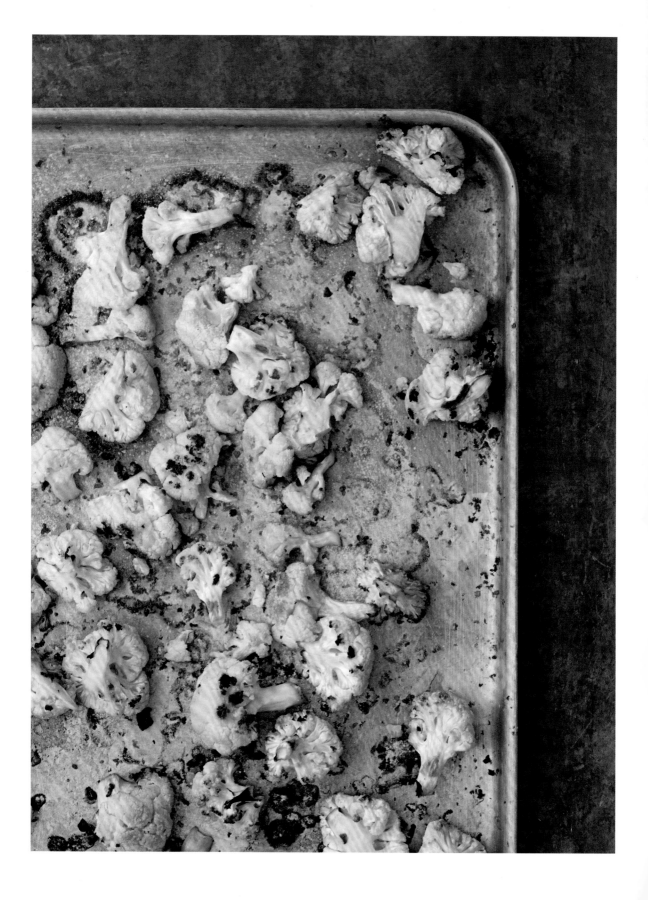

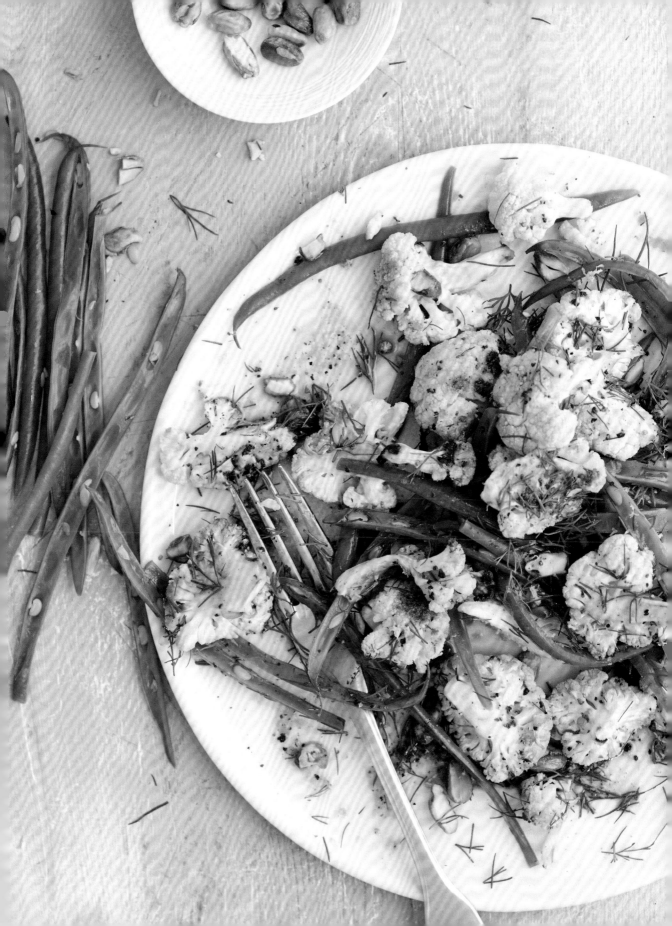

This is a great one-pot wonder you can chuck into the oven
and leave while you enjoy your favourite programme or have a bath.
Also a great one to make lots of and freeze in single-portion sizes
for a rainy day when you have no food in the fridge.

SERVES 3–4

curried aubergine

Preheat the oven to 180°C/160°C fan/gas mark 4.

In a flameproof casserole dish over a medium heat, melt the coconut oil and then add the onion and garlic, vegetable bouillon powder, mustard seeds and garam masala. Sauté for 1 minute before adding 60ml water and continuing to sauté for a further 2 minutes.

Add the tomatoes, another 100ml water and the tamari and continue to sauté for a further 2 minutes. Then add the aubergine and sauté for 3–4 minutes.

Finally, add the coconut milk and bay leaves and put the pan into the oven for 30 minutes.

When you take the pan out of the oven, the sauce should have reduced and be nice and thick. Stir through the fresh spinach and coriander and add a squeeze of lime, if you like. Serve the curry just as it is, or with some wild or brown rice.

1 tsp coconut oil
½ large or 1 small red onion, finely chopped
1 large clove garlic, finely chopped
½ tsp vegetable bouillon powder
1 tsp black mustard seeds
2 tsp garam masala
250g tomatoes, roughly chopped
2 tsp tamari
200g aubergine, cut into 2cm cubes
400ml coconut milk
2 bay leaves
60g fresh spinach
15g coriander, roughly chopped
a squeeze of lime (optional)

>>●

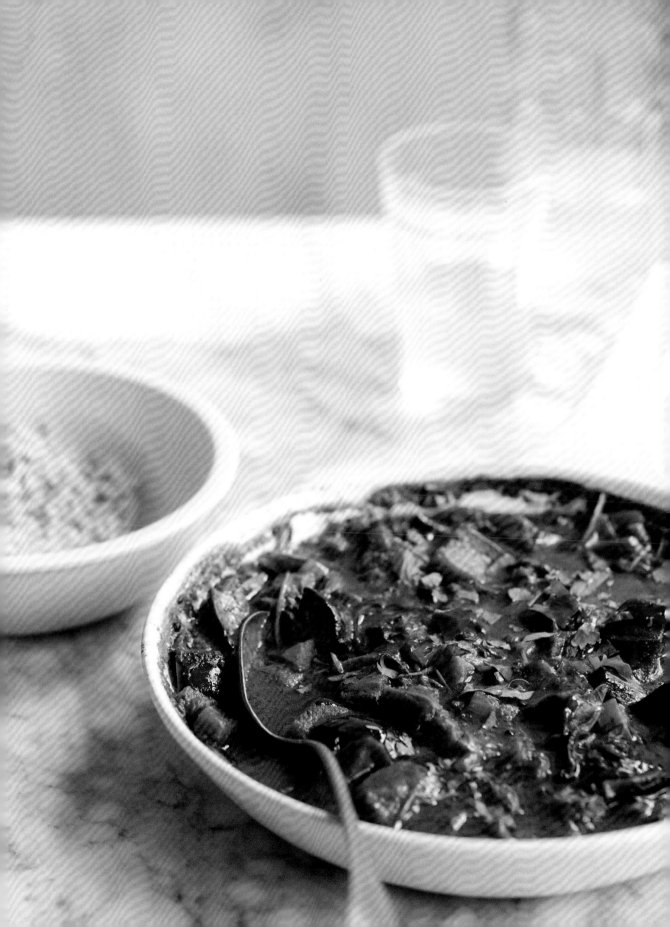

Stir-fry is the king of quick dinners, and this one has so much flavour it will have your taste buds singing till bedtime! Use the dressing for other dishes as well – it makes a wonderful alternative to a normal salad dressing. If you can't find fresh shiitake, you can use portobello or dried shiitake and soak them to rehydrate. If you are not a fan of spicy chilli, just add less or none.

SERVES 1–2

shiitake stir-fry

Melt the coconut oil in a frying pan and add the garlic, ginger, chilli and spring onions and cook over a medium heat for 2 minutes.

Add the shiitake mushrooms with the tamari and sauté for another minute.

Add 125ml water, the pak choi and cabbage and stir for 2 minutes. Add the radishes, stir in the chopped coriander and take off the heat.

Make the dressing, pour over the stir-fry and enjoy.

1 tbsp coconut oil
1 clove garlic, finely sliced
2–3cm piece of root ginger, finely chopped
2–3cm piece of chilli, finely diced
2 spring onions, sliced at an angle
120g shiitake mushrooms, sliced
1 tbsp tamari
150g pak choi
120g Savoy cabbage
100g radishes, cut in quarters
15g coriander, chopped

for the coconut dressing:
1 tbsp desiccated coconut
zest and juice of ½ lime
1 tbsp walnut or sesame oil

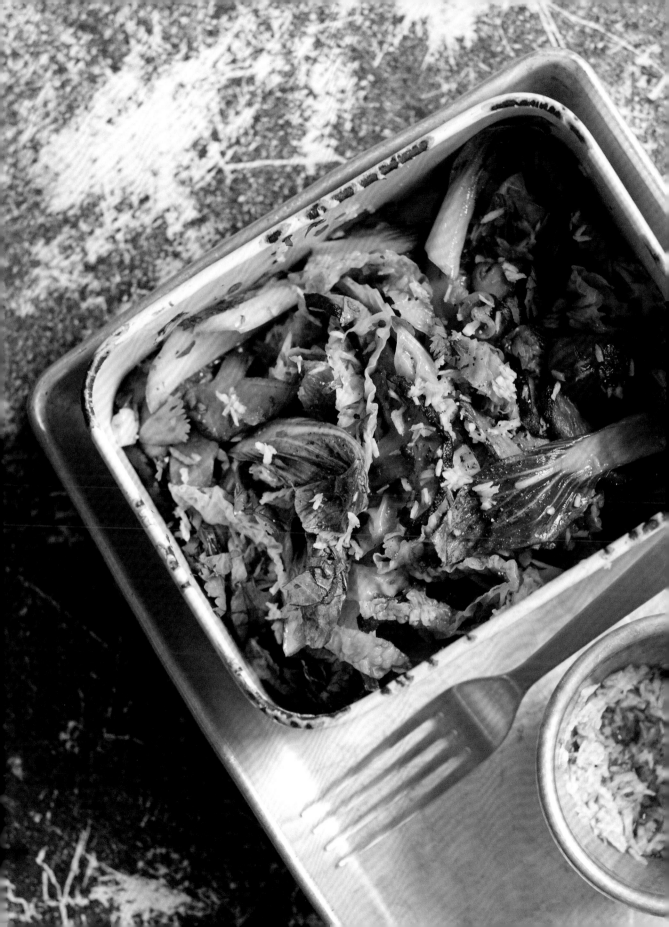

Crunchy and tasting just like the real deal, this tacos recipe is one not to miss. The tacos have become a staple in our home now and we bake them to order or in advance and have them all the time. The batter is so quick to make and you can also use it for a gluten-free wrap for the kids and big kids to take to work. In this case, don't put the tacos in the oven – simply wrap around a salad or my Sweet potato falafels (see page 148) for a healthy home-made lunch.

MAKES 4–5 TACOS

oven-baked gluten-free tacos *and* wraps

Preheat the oven to 170°C/150°C fan/gas mark 3. Remove one of the wire shelves as you will need it to drape your tacos over the bars so they dry into that classic U-shape.

Put the flour and salt into a bowl. Make a well in the middle, pour in 250ml water and mix together. Beat the egg in a separate bowl and then add to the flour and water until you have a thick batter.

Heat a good non-stick pan (mine is 30cm) and heat a small amount of sunflower oil spreading it over the surface. Ladle some batter into the pan and very quickly spread it out thinly to the edges by tilting the pan. Leave to cook, and as soon as it starts to bubble, lift around the edges and is golden underneath, flip it over and cook the other side. This should take 2 minutes on each side. Repeat until you have used up all the batter.

Put the wire shelf back into the preheated oven so it is sticking out of the door. Hang each taco over two wires next to each other. Once they are all hanging, push them down on the top so that they form a nice flat edge and straighten the sides so they are not too wide apart.

Carefully push the shelf into the oven and bake the tacos for 20 minutes until crisp. Meanwhile, make your fillings.

200g gluten-free plain flour
¼ tsp Himalayan pink salt
1 egg
sunflower oil, for frying

for the salsa:
345g vine tomatoes
15g coriander
juice of 1 lime
Himalayan pink salt

for the peppers:
1 tsp sunflower oil
1 red pepper, sliced
1 tbsp pomegranate molasses
1 tsp apple cider vinegar
a pinch of cayenne pepper

for the black beans:
1 tbsp sunflower oil
¼ tsp ground cumin
240g black beans
a pinch of paprika
avocado slices, for serving

＊

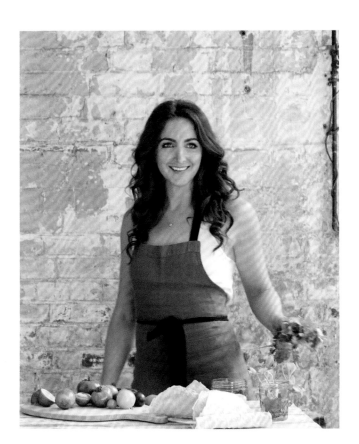

To make the salsa, whizz the tomatoes and coriander in a food processor, or chop finely by hand. Mix in the lime juice and salt. Transfer to a serving bowl.

For the peppers, put the sunflower oil into a pan with the sliced red pepper, pomegranate molasses, apple cider vinegar and cayenne pepper and sauté for 2–3 minutes. Add 60ml water and leave to be absorbed for another 2 minutes. Transfer to a serving bowl.

For the black beans, put the sunflower oil and cumin into a pan and leave on the heat for 1–2 minutes until the oil starts to sizzle. Add the beans and their liquid, then the paprika and stir for 2–3 minutes on a high heat until the liquid is reduced by half. Transfer to a serving bowl.

Carefully lift the tacos off the oven shelf and place on a platter on the table. Take care, as the tacos are crisp and crack easily.

To assemble, spoon a little of all the different accompaniments into your taco and top with the avocado slices. Enjoy with a napkin to hand!

✱

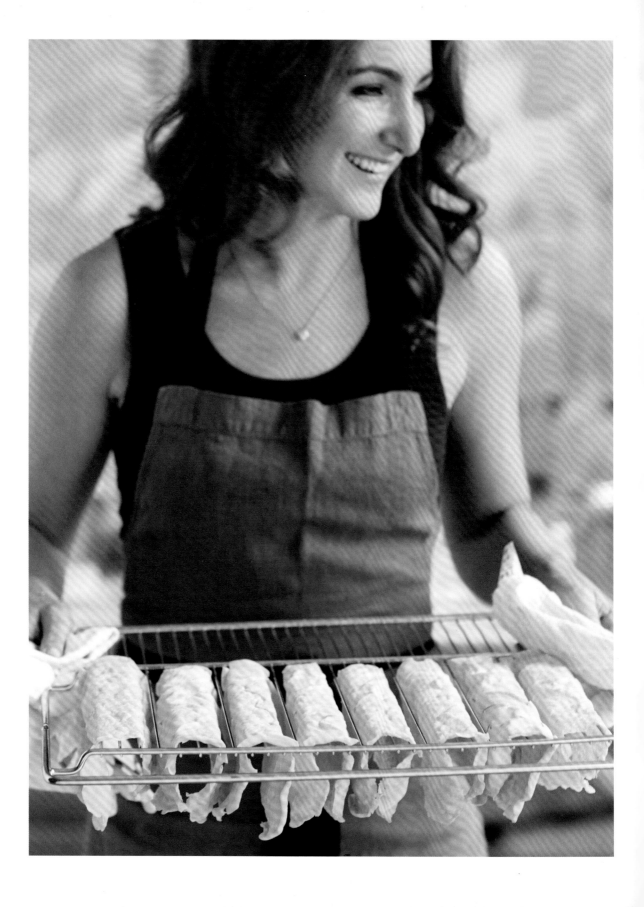

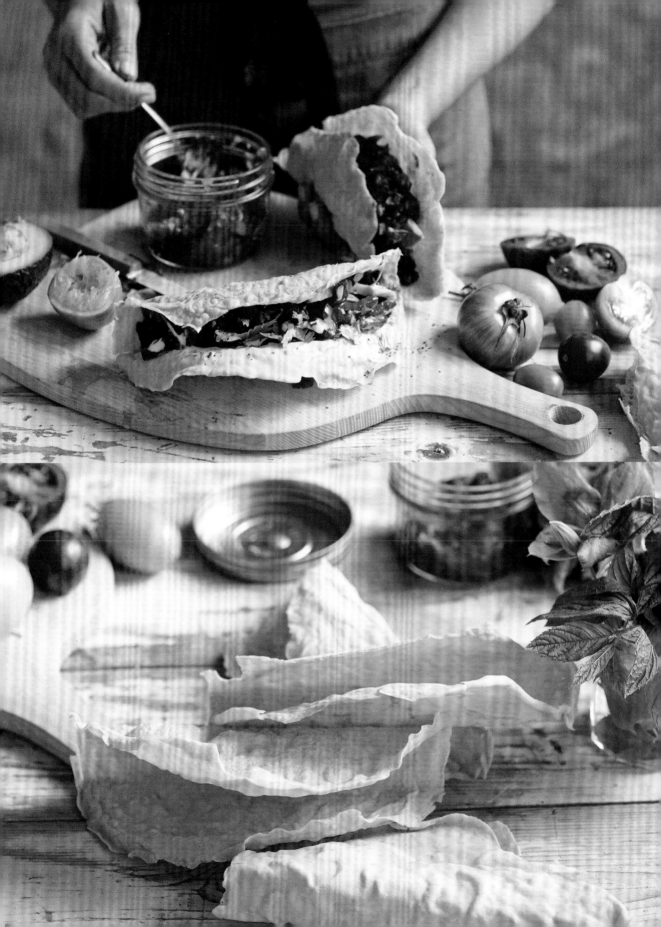

There really is nothing more satisfying than making a frittata.
It is always my fail-safe option if I need a quick dinner or
something to batch cook and keep in the fridge. Mr B loves it
too and requests it quite a lot for dinner! You don't have to
stick to the veg below – you can use pretty much anything
you have in your fridge – but do use the seasoning.

SERVES 4

leftovers duck egg frittata

Preheat the oven to 170°C/150°C fan/gas mark 3.

Beat together the eggs, salt, pepper, cumin and garlic in a bowl,
then add the rest of the vegetables and crumbled feta.

Heat the oil in a 20cm non-stick ovenproof frying pan for 1
minute. If you don't have a pan that small, you can use a larger
one, in which case the frittata will be thinner and take slightly
less time to cook. Add the egg mixture, placing the broccoli on
the top but making sure it's covered with the egg mixture or it
will burn when you put it in the oven. Leave to cook for 6
minutes so that the edges are firm.

Put the whole pan into the oven for 10 minutes or until there is
no liquid egg visible. Take out, remembering to use a cloth
around the handle – I have burnt my hand so many times!

Eat hot with a wonderful fresh salad, or set aside to cool, then
store in a sealed plastic container in the fridge for up to 4 days.

6 duck eggs or 8 large hen
   eggs
¼ tsp Himalayan pink salt
¼ tsp freshly ground black
   pepper
¼ tsp ground cumin
1 clove garlic, grated
20g fennel, shaved
30g cauliflower, shaved
50g Tenderstem broccoli,
   sliced lengthways
90g roasted sweet potato
   (130g raw sweet potato,
   peeled and roughly
   chopped) (see page 12)
40g feta cheese, crumbled
1 tsp sunflower oil

❯   1+2

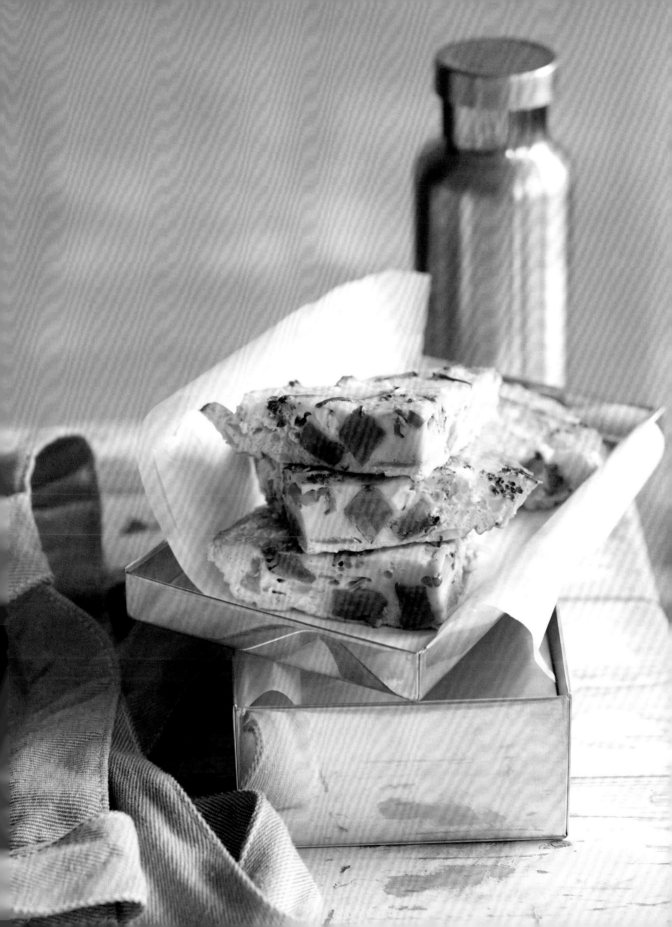

Quick, simple and packed full of protein. This is a great portable
recipe for eating after a workout and will give you loads of
energy for the rest of the day. I also like this with some fresh spinach
leaves or rocket to fill it out a bit and get in some extra greens!
Delicious with chargrilled broccoli on the side.

SERVES 2

creamy tahini lentils
with drippy boiled eggs

To boil the eggs, put them in a pan of boiling water for 7 minutes. Run them under cold water and peel the shells off.

Add the dill and mint to the Puy lentils with the lemon zest and a pinch of pepper.

Make the dressing by either blitzing up all the ingredients along with 5 tablespoons water in a blender, or whisking with a fork in a cup.

Drizzle the tahini dressing over the lentils, slice the eggs in half and place on top. Garnish with a little more pepper and a few fresh mint leaves.

2 eggs
15g dill, roughly chopped
5g mint, roughly chopped, plus extra leaves to garnish
240g cooked Puy lentils (120g uncooked weight) (see page 13); packets of precooked lentils also work brilliantly
zest of 1 lemon
freshly ground black pepper
fresh mint, to garnish

for the tahini dressing:
3 tbsp tahini
juice of ½ lemon
a pinch of Himalayan pink salt

❯ 1+2

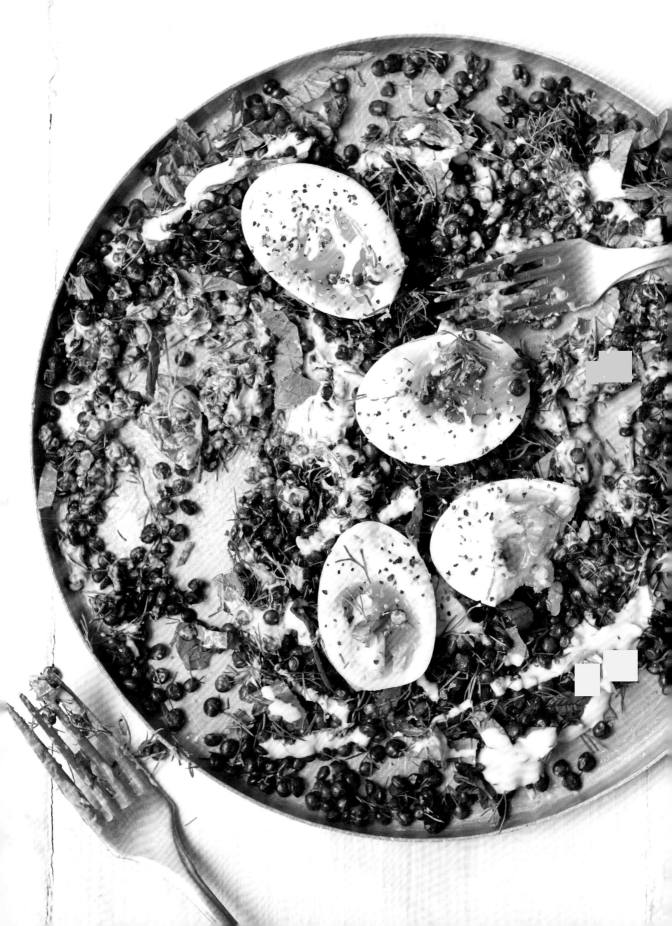

Stews are so comforting and this is a great one you can put together and then leave simmering away while you put your feet up or put the kids to bed. You can add different root vegetables from those listed, and if you have pre-roasted beetroot and celeriac, you can use them and the dish will take literally 10 minutes!

SERVES 2

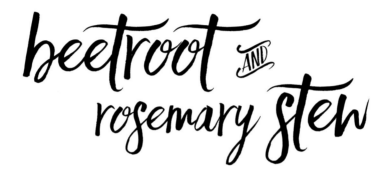

beetroot and rosemary stew

Sauté the onion, garlic and celery in the sunflower oil in a pan over a medium heat for 2 minutes. Add 1 tablespoon water, the salt and pepper and continue to sauté until the water has evaporated.

Next add the beetroot, celeriac, rosemary and bouillon powder and stir until coated. Add another 1 tablespoon water and continue to sauté for another 2 minutes.

Add 500ml water to the pan (250ml if using cooked beetroot and celeriac) and leave to simmer over a gentle heat for 30–35 minutes or until the beetroot is soft and the liquid has reduced to a nice thick sauce. If the beetroot and celeriac are already cooked, you can reduce the cooking time to 10 minutes.

Stir through the spinach until wilted, then stir in the parsley, dill and lemon juice. Remove the sprig of rosemary and enjoy!

1 red onion, sliced
2 cloves garlic, roughly chopped
35g celery, roughly chopped
2 tsp sunflower oil
¼ tsp Himalayan pink salt
a generous pinch of freshly ground black pepper
330g beetroot, peeled and chopped into 3cm chunks, or 250g cooked beetroot (see page 12)
250g celeriac, peeled and chopped into 3cm chunks, or 175g cooked celeriac (see page 12)
1 large sprig of rosemary
1 tsp vegetable bouillon powder
100g spinach
15g parsley, roughly chopped
15g dill, roughly chopped
juice of ½ lemon

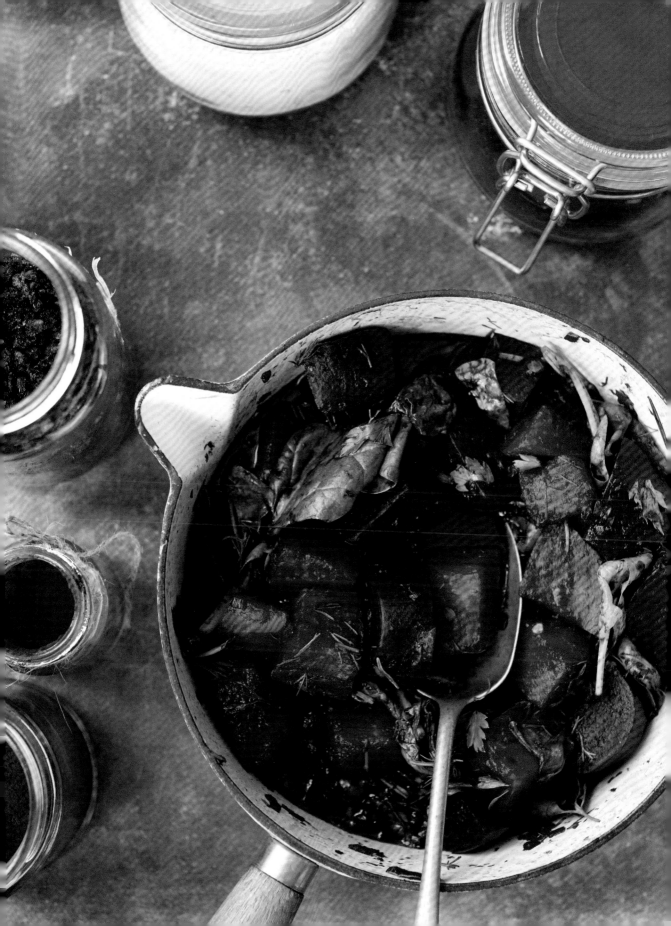

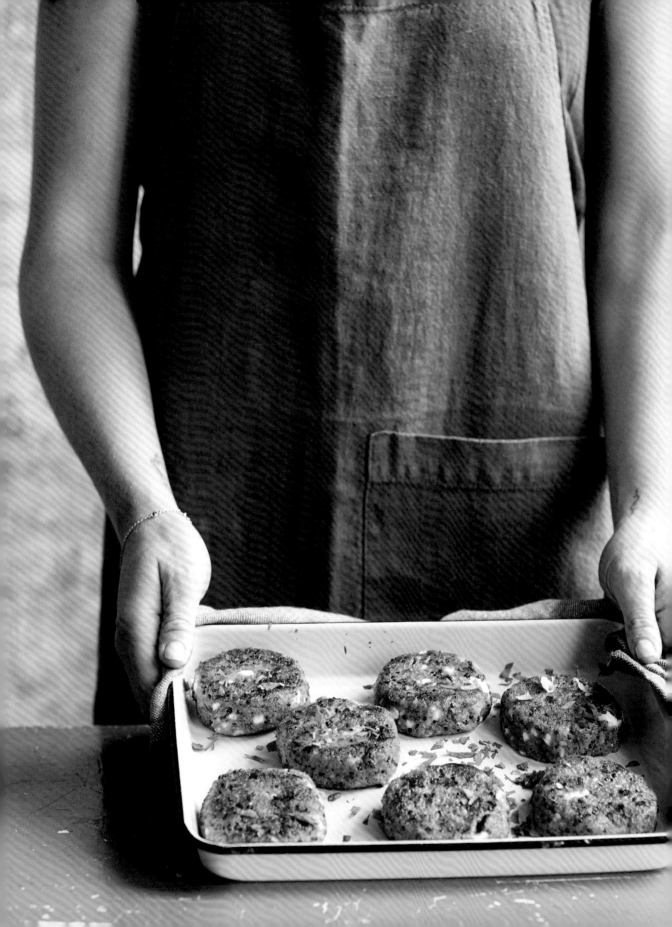

This is *the* perfect dish to rustle up if you have nailed your Sunday night prep. All you need to do is grab your precooked quinoa and roasted root veg from the fridge, throw in a couple of other ingredients and you are pretty much done. The whole process should take you no longer than 20 minutes, and you will be left with a completely delicious and satisfying dinner. You can also make these cakes with just sweet potato or butternut squash if needs be.

SERVES 3-4

root vegetable, quinoa AND feta cakes

200g precooked quinoa (110g uncooked quinoa) (see page 12)

130g roasted sweet potato (200g raw sweet potato, roasted whole) (see page 12)

130g roasted butternut squash (200g raw butternut squash, peeled and chopped) (see page 12)

130g feta cheese, crumbled

¼ tsp ground cumin

1 small clove garlic, grated

25g gluten-free plain flour

12g parsley, roughly chopped

a generous pinch of Himalayan pink salt and freshly ground black pepper

2 tsp sunflower oil

Preheat the oven to 180°C/160°C fan/gas mark 4.

Put your quinoa, sweet potato flesh and butternut squash into a food processor and blend until almost smooth – it's nice to keep a few chunks of the vegetables in there.

Transfer to a bowl and mix in all the remaining ingredients except for the sunflower oil.

Heat the sunflower oil in a frying pan over a medium heat. Shape the mixture into 6–8 little cakes and toast in the pan for just a minute on each side until golden.

Transfer to a baking tray and bake in the oven for 10 minutes until heated through.

Serve with a simple salad and lemony dressing.

1+2 >

This is such a zesty and vibrant-tasting salad, and the dressing is one you can use for anything to taste delicious. You can also make this recipe with griddled courgettes if you don't have any aubergine at home.

SERVES 2

griddled aubergine miso salad

Heat a griddle pan (or normal frying pan) over a medium heat. Put the aubergine into a bowl with the sunflower oil and salt and toss them around with your hands so each slice is lightly coated.

Cover the griddle pan in an even layer of the aubergine (you might need to do this in two batches) and griddle on each side for about 2 minutes until you start to get lovely charred marks. Transfer to a clean bowl and cook any remaining aubergine in the same way.

Meanwhile, make the dressing by whisking all of the ingredients together with 3 tablespoons water until nice and smooth.

Stir the quinoa into the aubergine. Pour in the dressing and mix well.

Boil the kettle, put the spinach in a sieve and pour the boiling water over so it wilts. Add the wilted spinach to the quinoa mixture.

Top the dressed aubergine with the lime zest, sesame seeds, coriander, spring onions and chilli and stir once again.

280g aubergine, sliced into circles
1 tbsp sunflower oil
a pinch of Himalayan pink salt
190g precooked quinoa (100g uncooked quinoa) (see page 12)
70g fresh spinach leaves
zest of ½ lime
1 tsp sesame seeds
25g coriander, roughly chopped
1 large or 2 small spring onions, finely chopped
½ red chilli, finely chopped

for the miso dressing:
1½ tbsp brown rice miso
1½ tsp sesame oil
juice of ½ lime

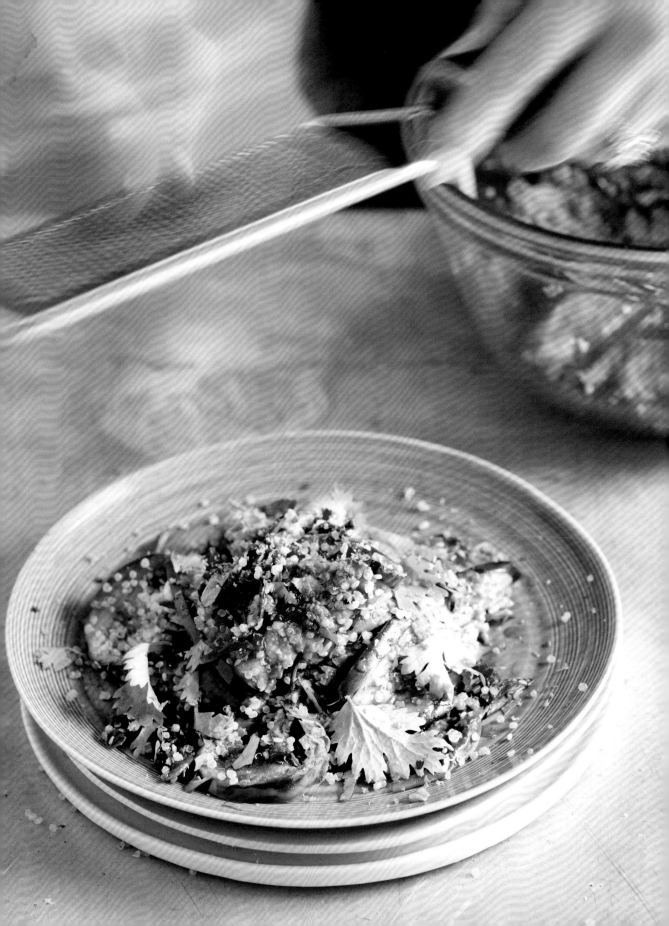

I have had a slight obsession with lemony and salty cucumber for some time now, so I had to write a recipe for it so you can jump on my bandwagon! I love this salad – it is so fresh and zesty, perfect as an accompaniment or side dish.

SERVES 2

smashed salted cucumber, mint and avocado

Cut the small cucumbers into quarters and put into a freezer bag with the salt and lemon juice. Get a rolling pin and bash the outside of the bag so the cucumbers smash up (don't go crazy thinking of your ex-boyfriend and massacre them – just enough so they are slightly broken on the edges). Shake the bag so that the salt and lemon juice are covering the cucumbers evenly. Leave for 15 minutes, or longer if you have the time.

Cut the avocado into slices and arrange on a plate. Add chunks of feta, whole fresh mint leaves and the smashed cucumber. Drizzle with the olive oil and serve as a side dish, or add salad leaves for a main.

3 small cucumbers
a large pinch of Himalayan pink salt
juice of ½ lemon
1 avocado, peeled and stone removed
150g feta cheese
15g mint (fresh whole leaves)
1 tbsp olive oil

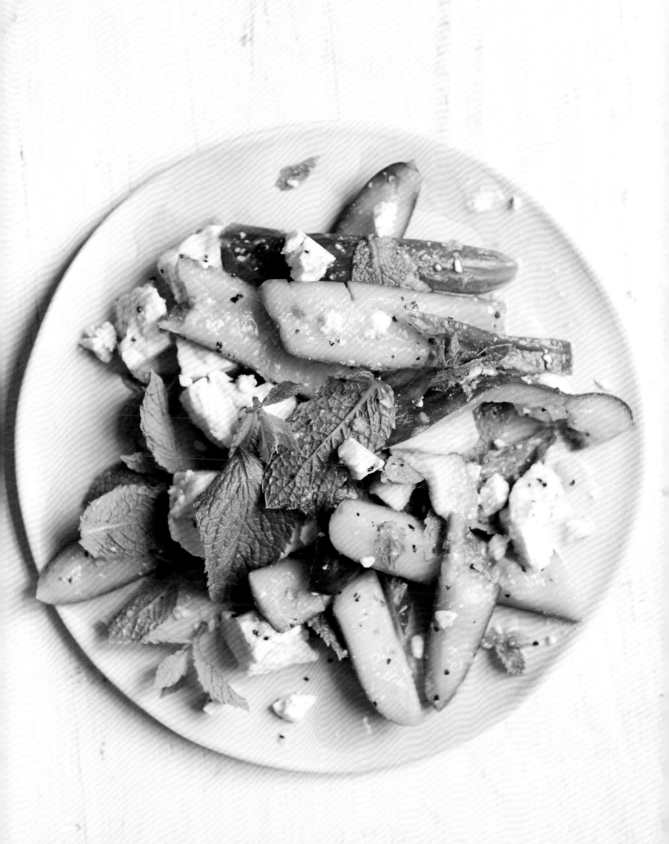

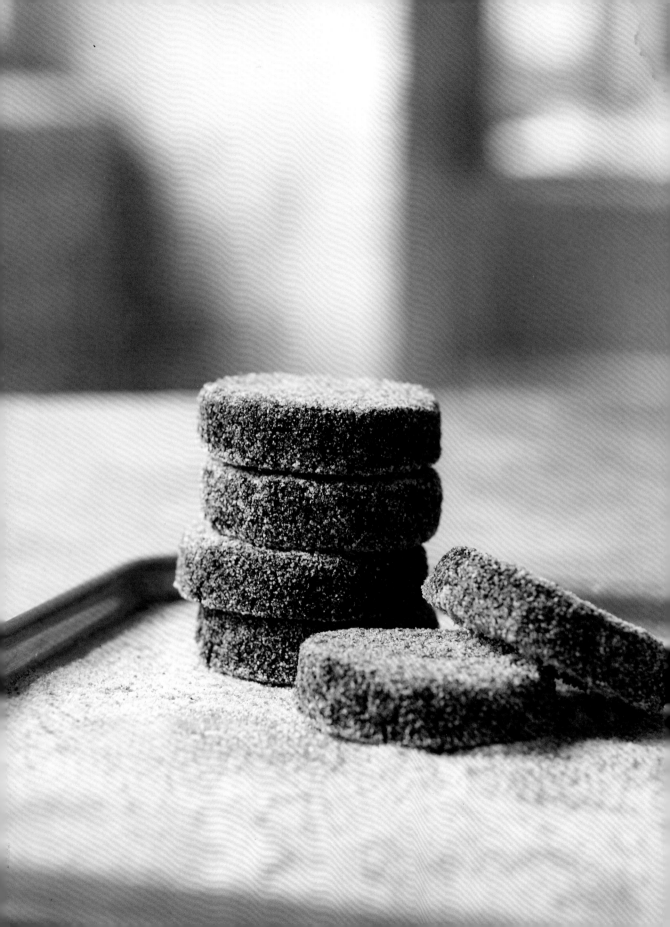

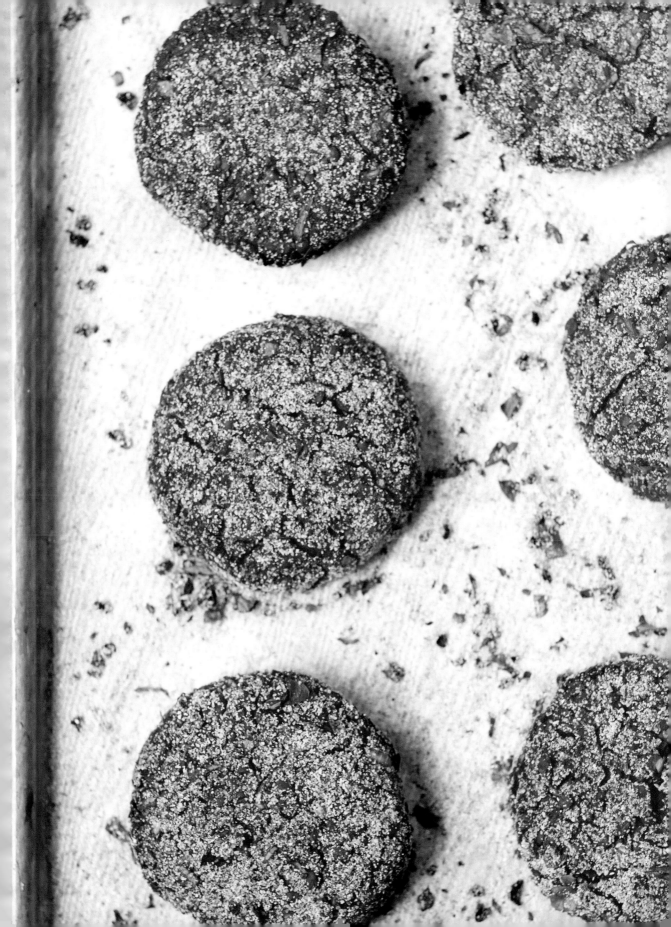

If you want a burger that holds together and sits well between a bun, this is one to try. The longer you leave the polenta to sit in the mixture uncooked, the firmer the burgers will become. Great for a picnic, especially if served with caramelised onions in a gluten-free burger bun.

MAKES 6 BURGERS

beetroot burgers

Preheat the oven to 180°C/160°C fan/gas mark 4.

Place all of the ingredients except for the parsley in a food processor and gently blitz until the lentils break down a little and the mixture starts to come together. Don't over-blitz, though, as you want to retain some of the texture.

Scoop the mixture out of the food processor and into a bowl and stir through the chopped parsley.

Divide the mixture into six equal pieces and shape into burgers with your hands. You can make the burgers in advance up to this point.

Pour some additional polenta onto a plate and sprinkle over the burgers, being careful to sprinkle round the sides too.

Bake the burgers in the oven on a baking tray for 15–20 minutes until warmed through and a little crispy on the outside.

2 spring onions, very finely chopped
1 large clove garlic, grated
½ tsp ground coriander
250g cooked Puy lentils (125g uncooked weight) (see page 13); packets of precooked lentils also work brilliantly
230g grated raw beetroot
¼ tsp Himalayan pink salt
¼ tsp freshly ground black pepper
zest and juice of ½ lemon
3 tbsp polenta, plus extra for rolling out
15g parsley, chopped

1+2

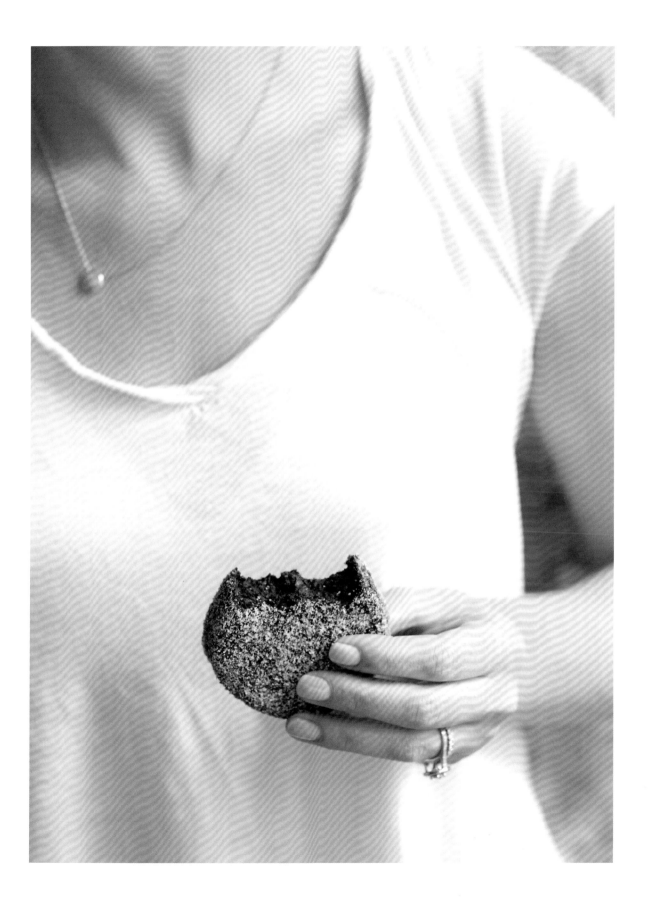

Having these stock cubes in the freezer makes life quick and easy as you don't need to use onion, garlic or spices when you are cooking as it's all in the stock. Make up a batch and freeze in your ice-cube tray so you can whip up a soup, stock or stir-fry without the hassle of chopping.

MAKES 24–28 ICE CUBES

iced stock cubes

Put the onion into a blender with 500ml hot water and the rest of the ingredients and blend until it becomes a textured liquid.

Pour into ice-cube trays and put in the freezer for when you need them. Just add a little water when you are cooking them out as the flavour is quite concentrated.

100g onion, diced

2 cloves garlic, grated

1 tbsp ground cumin

1 tbsp ground coriander

1 tsp mustard seeds

2 tbsp sunflower or coconut oil

3 tbsp vegetable bouillon powder

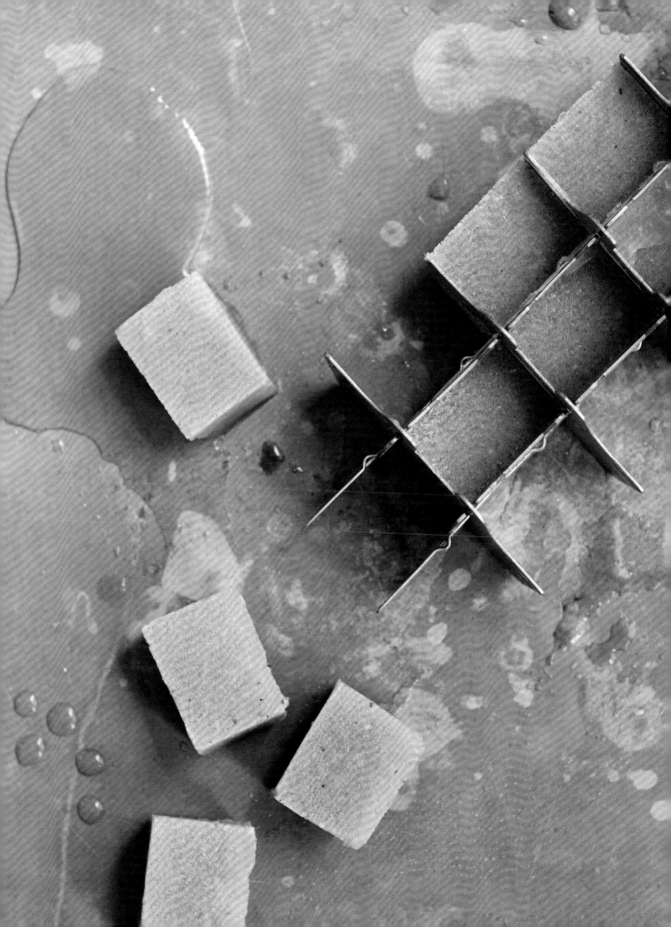

This is such a spring salad for me and so full of flavour.
I love using grapefruit in salads as they are both sweet and
zesty. If you don't have time to cook wild rice, you can
use quinoa or any other gluten-free grain instead, or go
grain-free if you fancy a really light dish.

SERVES 2

roasted radish and citrus salad

Preheat the oven to 170°C/150°C fan/gas mark 3.

Put the whole radishes and asparagus spears on a baking tray, drizzle with the sunflower oil and put into the oven for 10 minutes.

Boil a pan of water, add the salt and blanch the green beans in it for 3 minutes. Drain and run them under cold water straight away.

Separate the chicory leaves and put into a bowl with the green beans.

Segment the grapefruit by cutting off the peel and slicing between each side of the membrane with a sharp knife. Add the segments to the bowl.

Add the spring onion, parsley, wild rice, baked radishes and asparagus to the rest of the salad ingredients.

Make the dressing by putting all the ingredients into a blender and blitzing until smooth.

Mix the dressing through the salad and serve.

80g radishes
100g asparagus
1 tsp sunflower oil
1 tbsp Himalayan pink salt
100g green beans
1 chicory
1 grapefruit
1 spring onion, thinly sliced at an angle
10g parsley, roughly chopped
195g precooked wild rice (80g uncooked wild rice) (see page 12)

for the parsley dressing:
10g parsley
50ml olive oil
40ml apple cider vinegar
juice of ½ lemon
a pinch of Himalayan pink salt

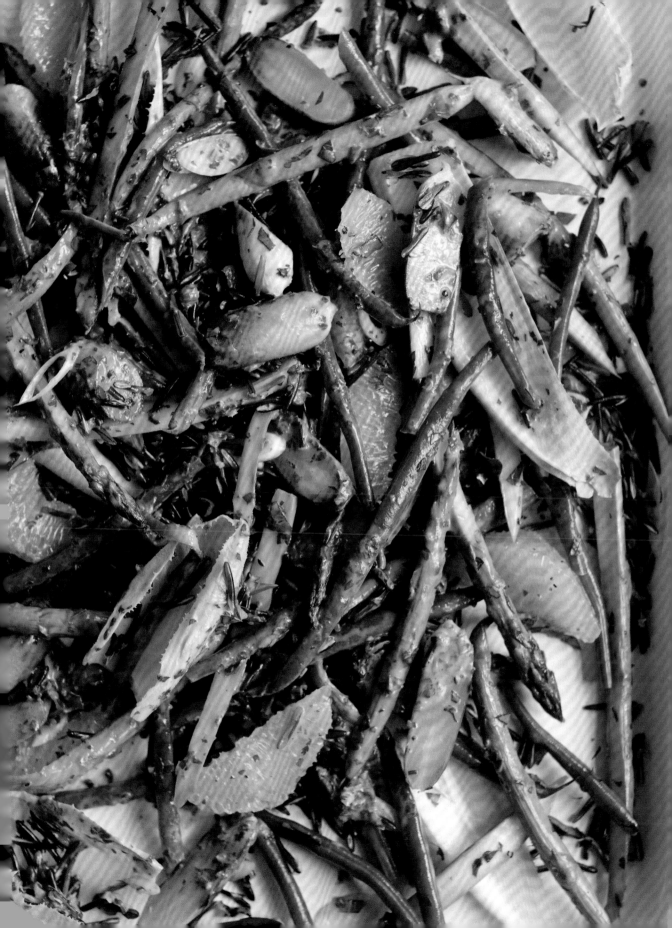

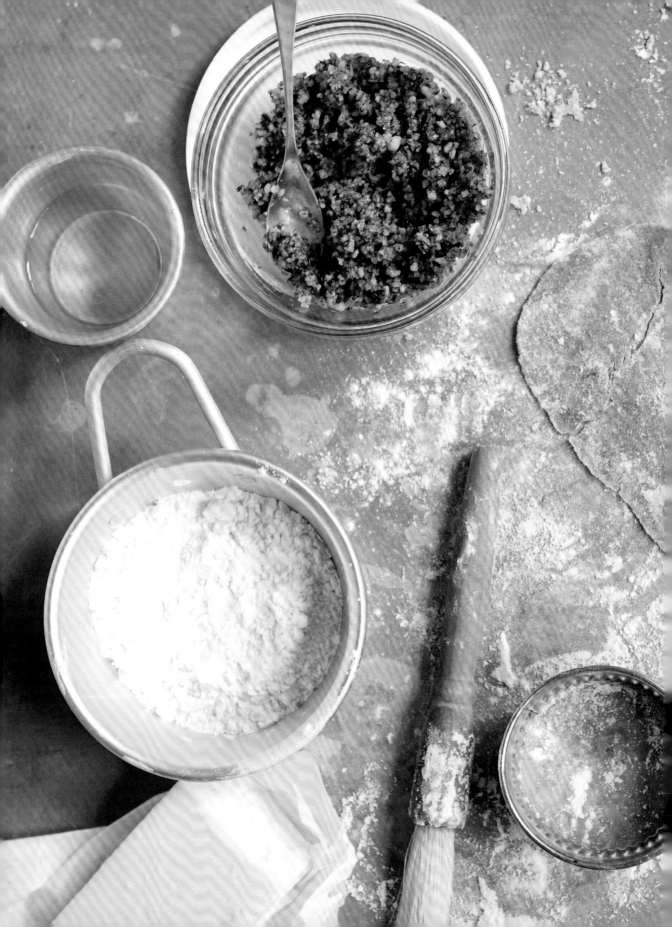

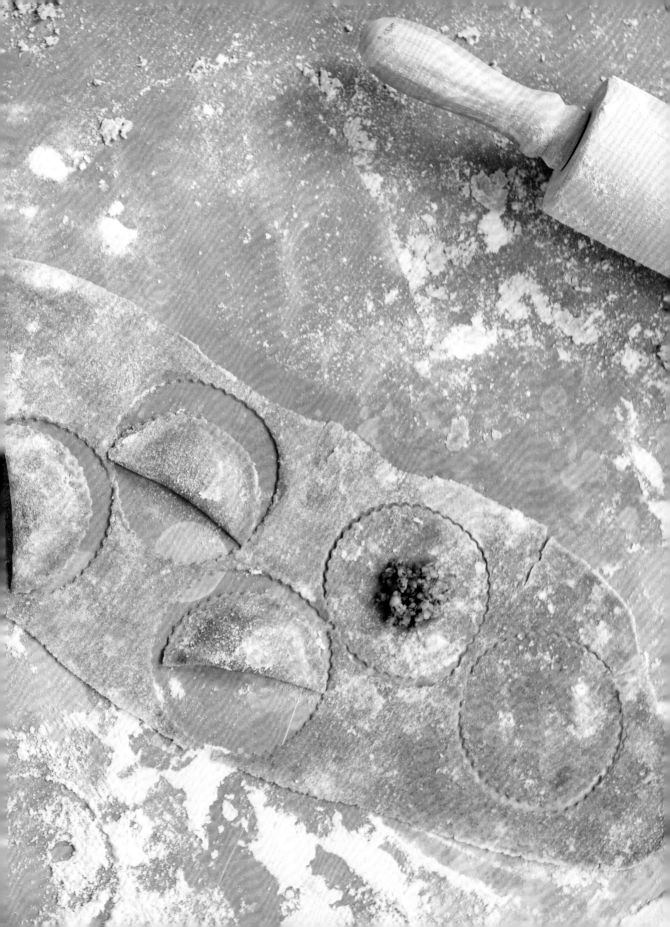

When I was developing this recipe, I timed myself making the whole thing and it took me 35 minutes start to finish. I have also included a tagliatelle option for those of you who might want an even quicker recipe. Essentially, though, I wanted to show you that making your own pasta does not have to be a difficult or time-consuming task. No laborious winding through pasta machines and hanging over your laundry rack. Just rolling, shaping, cooking. The ravioli freeze really well, so you can pop them out of the freezer and into a pan of boiling water for an even quicker dinner. I have used my frozen pesto cubes for the filling, but you can use any roasted vegetable made into a purée, and you can add some goats' cheese for added creaminess. Even my tapenade topping (see page 158) would work really well as a filling.

SERVES 2–3

buckwheat *and* pesto ravioli

Put the flour and salt into a bowl. Make a well in the centre and mix in the beaten egg. Keep mixing and it will become crumb-like. Add 2 teaspoons water, a teaspoon at a time. Bring the dough together and knead for a couple minutes on a well-floured surface – it will start to develop a lovely smooth texture.

Dampen a cloth and place it over the dough – this will stop it from drying out. Take a quarter of the mixture at a time and roll it out as thinly as you can without cracking (ideally 1mm thick). The thinner you get it, the softer your pasta will be when cooked.

Once rolled out, cut out circles with a 9cm cutter and repeat this over all the dough.

If you need to defrost the pesto cubes, put them into a saucepan with 60ml water and the oil and heat until it becomes a soft, thick paste. Grate in the goats' cheese with the fine side of the grater and dollop ½ teaspoon of the mixture into the middle of each pasta circle.

140g buckwheat flour
generous pinch of Himalayan pink salt
1 egg, beaten
2½ tsp olive oil
freshly ground black pepper

for the frozen filling:
6 frozen Perfect pesto cubes (see page 181)
1 tbsp sunflower oil
10g hard goats' cheese

for the fresh filling:
4 tbsp Perfect pesto (see page 181)
5mm cubes of hard goats' cheese or feta cheese (optional)

*

If you are using fresh pesto, just dollop ½ teaspoon into the middle of each circle. Top with a little chunk of cheese, if using.

Dip your finger into some cold water and run it around the edge of each circle. Fold into a half-moon shape and pinch the edges together to seal. Make sure there are no gaps or the filling will come out and the water will flood in when you cook them.

Bring a large pan of water to the boil, then add a pinch of salt and a teaspoon of the olive oil. When it is at a rolling boil, drop in the ravioli, being careful not to put too many in the pan at the same time as they might break. Cook for 8–10 minutes until soft.

Serve the ravioli with the remaining olive oil and black pepper and mix in the rest of the pesto to coat the outside.

tagliatelle

If you would rather opt to make tagliatelle, follow the method until the cutting stage. Instead of using the cutter, just slice the dough into long strips about 1cm wide. Drop into the pan of boiling water with a teaspoon of olive oil and a pinch of salt and cook for 4 minutes before draining. Stir through a generous dollop of pesto and serve with some lovely grated goats' cheese over the top.

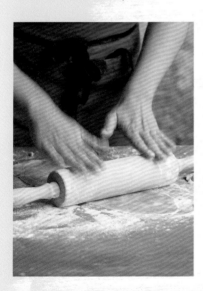
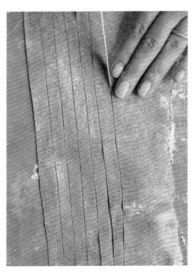
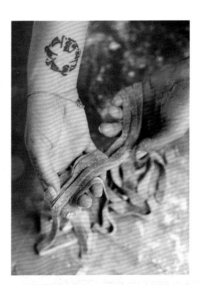

This is the most creamy and satisfying of all mash recipes.
Polenta is such a quick ingredient to cook with – it takes
literally 2 minutes to make and adds a really hearty sustenance
to dishes like this. I hate wasting veg, so if you have any celeriac left
over, just roast it as well and use for a wonderful root vegetable
salad. You can always make double and freeze it so you
always have delicious mash to tuck into.

SERVES 2–3

celeriac and polenta mash

Preheat the oven to 180°C/160°C fan/gas mark 4.

Put the celeriac into a roasting tray and sprinkle with the cumin and a teaspoon of the sunflower oil. Roast for 30 minutes until soft.

Meanwhile, put the onion and the remaining teaspoon of sunflower oil into a pan over a medium heat and sauté for 2 minutes until soft. Add 60ml water, the celery and the bouillon powder and continue to sauté for a further 4 minutes until it makes a wonderful thick stock.

Add 250ml water, the polenta and lemon zest and cook for 2–3 minutes, whisking continuously so as not to get any lumps. It will bubble and spit, so be careful.

Place the polenta and roasted celeriac in a food processor with the milk. Season well with salt and pepper and blend until completely smooth.

Serve the mash with sautéed mushrooms and lots of herbs, or use as a topping for a shepherd's pie or lentil bake.

315g raw celeriac, peeled and chopped into 2cm cubes
¼ tsp ground cumin
2 tsp sunflower oil
½ red onion, finely diced
½ stick celery, roughly chopped
½ tbsp vegetable bouillon powder
50g polenta
zest of ½ lemon
290ml milk
Himalayan pink salt and freshly ground black pepper

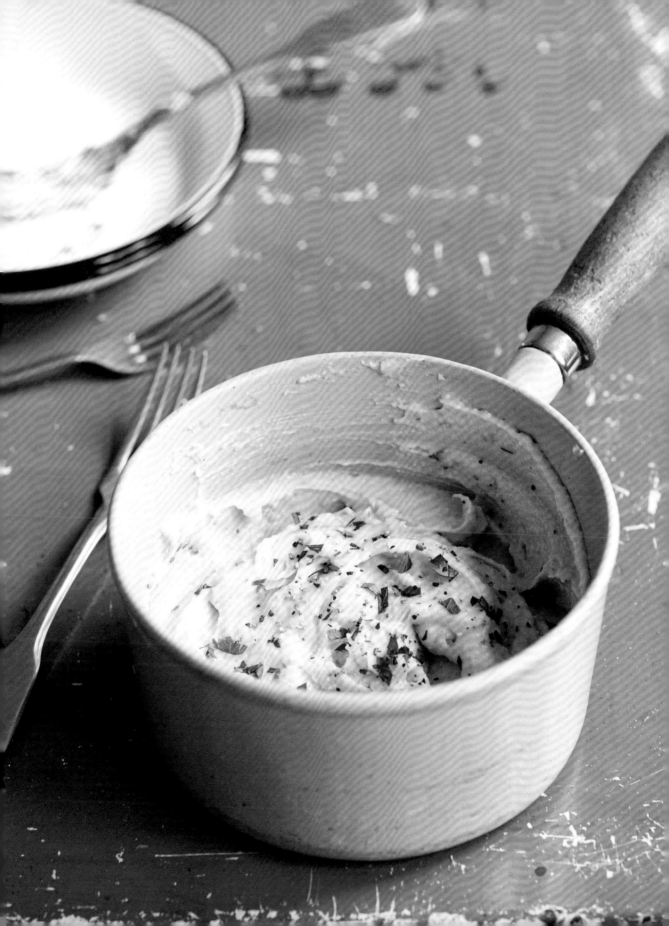

I love salads and this one is a favourite because it has so many hidden flavours in it. If you haven't got blackberries or they're out of season, you could use a different berry or even a juicy pear in the winter months.

SERVES 2

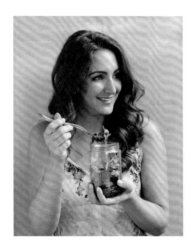

rice, blackberry and carrot salad

Layer the salad ingredients in a glass bowl or jar if you want the salad to look pretty.

Mix the dressing ingredients (apart from the zest) together in a glass and pour over the top of the salad. Sprinkle with the lime zest and serve. Or see page 21 for a great tip on transporting your salad dressing!

250g precooked wild or brown rice (100g uncooked rice) (see page 12)
60g blackberries
100g carrots, grated
60g courgettes, grated
5g mint leaves
10g dill, chopped
20g shelled pistachios

for the pomegranate molasses dressing:
1 tbsp mirin
2 tbsp olive oil
1 tbsp pomegranate molasses
a big pinch of Himalayan pink salt
juice and zest of 2 limes

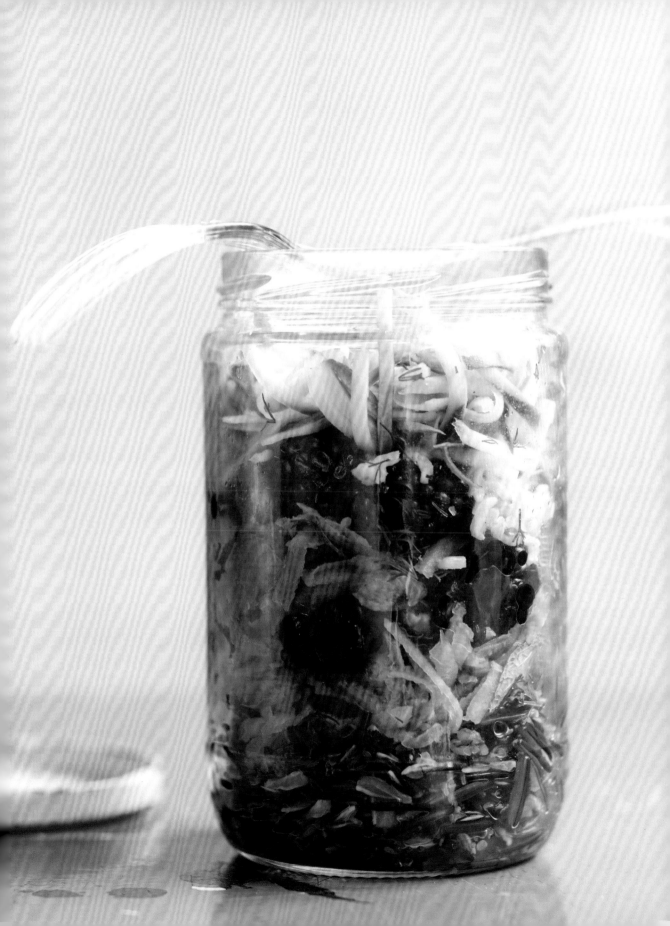

Currently one of my all-time favourite go-to Sunday
night dishes. I always roast sweet potatoes for the week
ahead, so this is a quick dish to rustle up and great to
take to work the next day for a healthy lunch.

SERVES 3–4

herbed sweet potato salad

Finely chop the broccoli florets so they look like seeds. Place in a bowl with the dill, mint, alfalfa sprouts, spinach leaves and cooled sweet potato. Add the remaining ingredients and a pinch of salt and pepper. Mix well and serve.

50g broccoli tops (florets without the stalks)
10g dill, roughly chopped
10g mint, roughly chopped
20g alfalfa sprouts
30g spinach or wild salad leaves
120g roasted sweet potato (190g raw sweet potato, quartered lengthways) (see page 12)
zest and juice of 1 lemon
1 tbsp olive oil
¼ tsp sumac
Himalayan pink salt and freshly ground black pepper

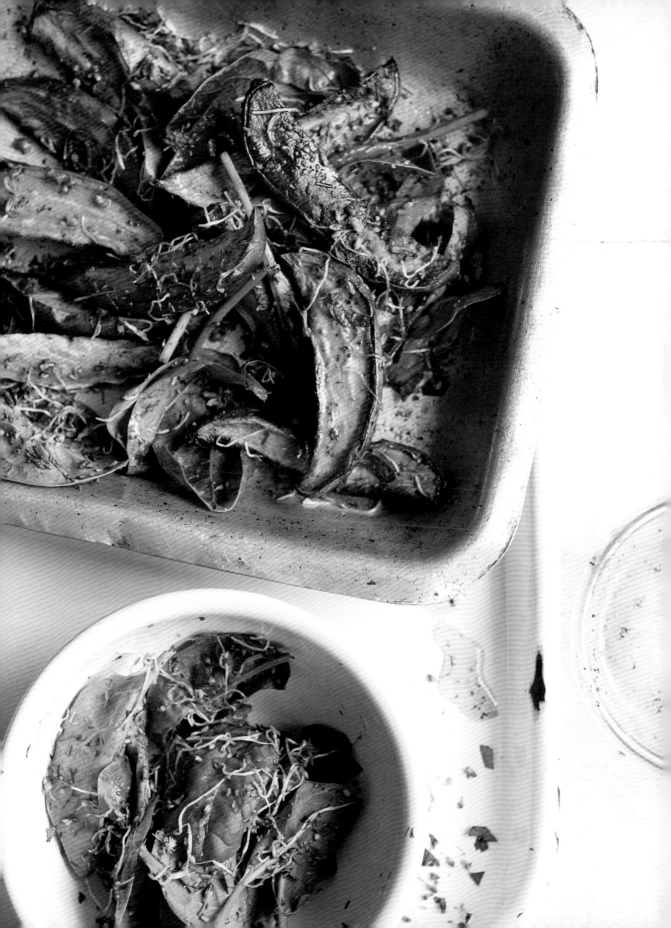

Aubergines can be really filling and meaty, and with the right flavours become slightly addictive. This dish is a great one to make at the weekend and use the following week, cold from the fridge, in a salad or perhaps to make a speedy version of the Griddled aubergine miso salad (see page 110).

SERVES 2

roasted aubergine
AND
onion seeds

Preheat the oven to 180°C/160°C fan/gas mark 4.

Slice the aubergine in half lengthways. Put the halves onto a baking tray, flesh side up.

Smear the garlic over the flesh of the aubergine, sprinkle evenly with the salt, cumin, nigella seeds and oil.

Put into the oven for 40–45 minutes until soft. Five minutes before the aubergine is done, sprinkle the spring onion over the top to cook. Season with pepper.

Serve as a side dish with a salad.

400g (1 large) aubergine
2 cloves garlic, crushed
¼ tsp Himalayan pink salt
¼ tsp ground cumin
¼ tsp nigella (onion) seeds
4 tbsp sunflower oil
2 spring onions, chopped
freshly ground black pepper

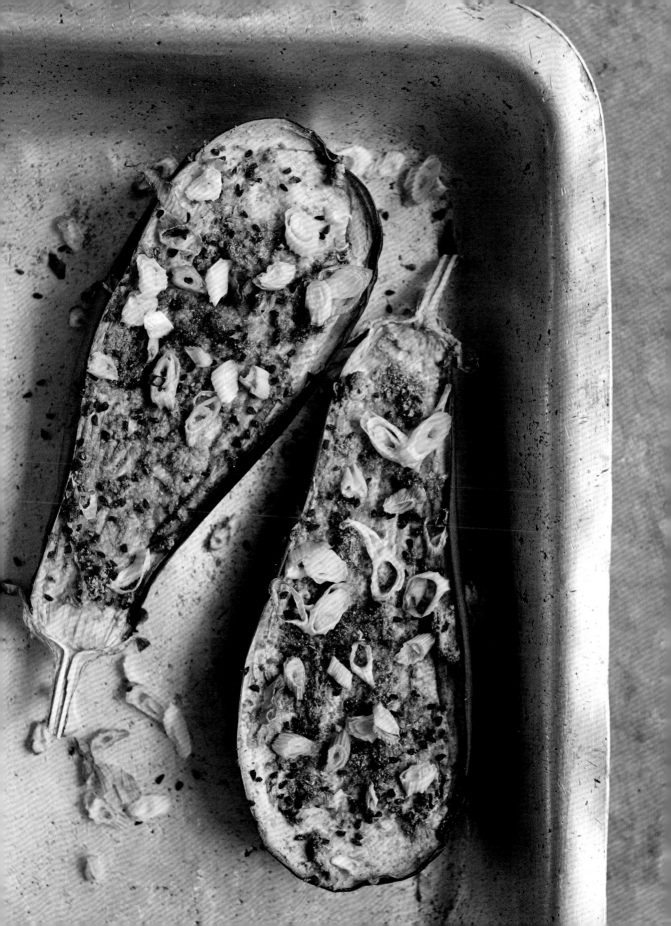

If you need a comfort food fix, this is the perfect dish to make. It's quick to pull together and then you can leave it to cook in the oven while you get on with other things. You can also reheat it, so it's perfect for a dinner party.

SERVES 3-4

moussaka

Preheat the oven to 180°C/160°C fan/gas mark 4.

Place the aubergine in a bowl and add 300ml water and ½ teaspoon of salt. Set aside for 10 minutes. This will help to draw out the water from the aubergine, which will in turn mean less cooking time for you!

Put the sunflower oil in a flameproof dish or roasting tray and sauté the onion over a medium heat with the garlic, cinnamon and cumin. After about 2 minutes, add 60ml water and continue to sauté for a further 2-3 minutes until the water has evaporated.

Add the tomatoes and pomegranate molasses and continue to sauté. After a further 2 minutes, add 125ml water, the bay leaf and rosemary and leave to simmer for 3 minutes. Drain the aubergine and add to the pan with another 500ml water and continue to cook until the liquid has thickened. This should take another 7-8 minutes.

Once the aubergine has softened, add the courgettes and stir through. Leave on the heat for 3-4 minutes to cook through, then add the chickpeas and season with a pinch of salt and pepper. Leave to simmer.

Meanwhile, make the topping. Put the feta and manchego in a bowl. Whisk in the egg, tahini, almond milk and some seasoning until thoroughly combined.

Pour the egg mixture over the top of the aubergine and bake in the oven for 25-30 minutes or until the topping is starting to bubble and turn golden brown.

130g aubergine, chopped into 2cm cubes
2 tbsp sunflower oil
½ red onion, roughly diced
2 cloves garlic, roughly chopped
1 tsp ground cinnamon
1 tsp ground cumin
350g tomatoes, roughly chopped
1 tsp pomegranate molasses
1 bay leaf
1 large sprig of rosemary
120g courgettes, cut into 1cm batons
230g cooked chickpeas (400g tin, drained)
Himalayan pink salt and freshly ground black pepper

for the topping:
70g feta cheese, crumbled
30g manchego or pecorino cheese, grated
1 egg
1 tsp tahini
125ml almond or other plant milk (bought or see page 52)

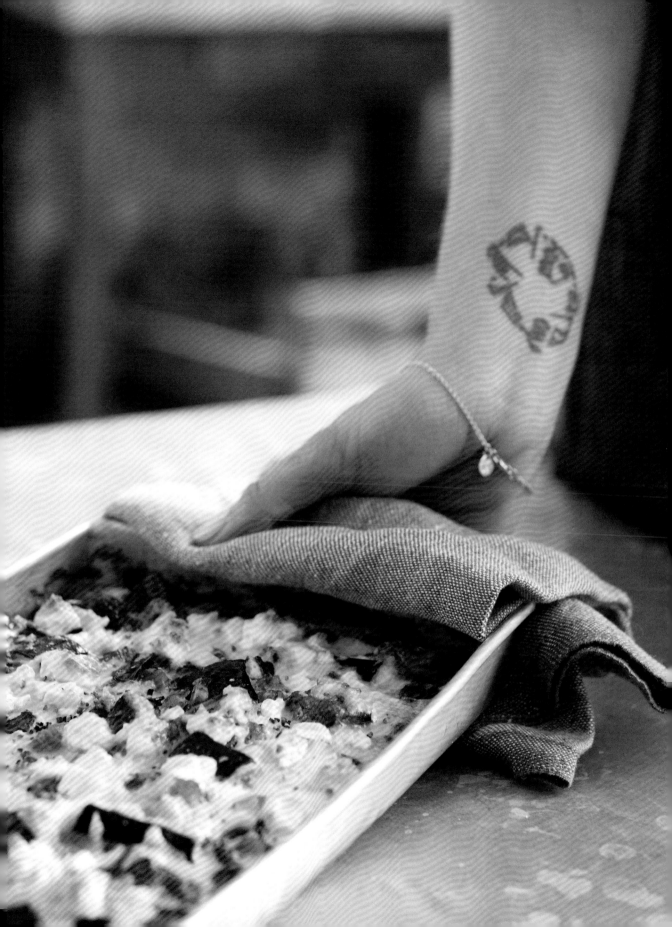

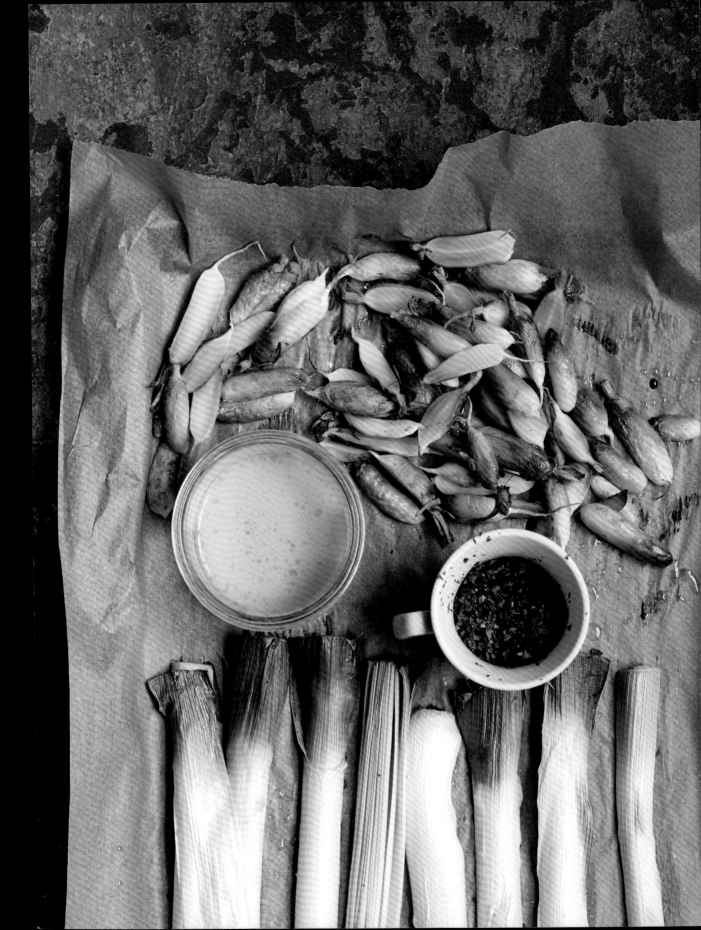

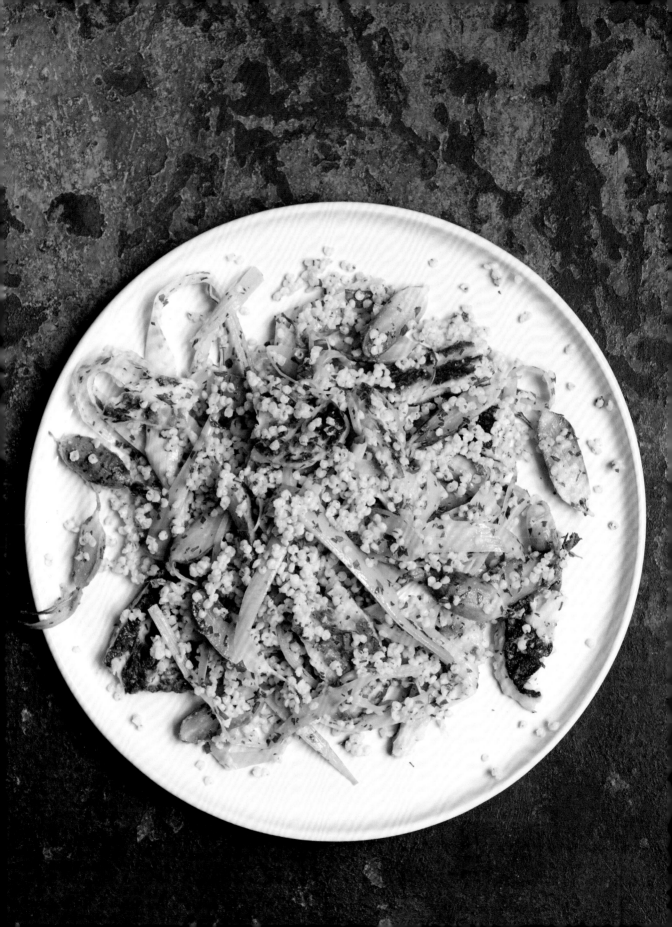

A wonderfully filling and fulfilling salad that can be created
so quickly, and even quicker if you have precooked millet.
I love millet as it is so nutty and versatile – you can
make porridge out of it and even burgers. Get to love
this new and exciting gluten-free grain.

SERVES 2-3

leek *and* halloumi millet salad

Preheat the oven to 170°C/150°C fan/gas mark 3.

Cut the leeks lengthways and put in a baking tray with the radishes. Pour the sunflower oil over the top and cook for 10–15 minutes until both are soft.

Evenly slice the halloumi and place in a frying pan over a medium heat. Cook for about 2–3 minutes on each side until golden.

Divide the millet between 2 or 3 plates and place the leeks on top. Cut the radishes in half and arrange them on top with the halloumi slices and chopped parsley.

Make the dressing by blitzing all the ingredients in a blender. Drizzle over the salad and serve.

4 small leeks (485g)
250g radishes
1 tsp sunflower oil
200g halloumi cheese
130g precooked millet (320g uncooked millet) (see page 12)
30g parsley, chopped

for the apple cider vinegar dressing:
juice of 1 lemon
3 tbsp olive oil
a pinch of Himalayan pink salt
1 tsp apple cider vinegar

1+2

This is that salad that bridges the gap between fresh summer
ingredients and classically English rainy days. Warm but super
bright and fresh. If you don't have baby gem lettuce, iceberg lettuce
will work just as well. Similarly, if you don't have green beans,
try adding some peas. It's a pretty versatile dish, so have a
play with different ingredients.

SERVES 2

warm halloumi and mint salad

2 tsp coconut oil
1 clove garlic, thinly sliced
¼ tsp fennel seeds
160g halloumi, sliced
2 baby gem lettuces (250g)
¼ tsp Himalayan pink salt
200g green beans, topped
    and tailed
10g mint, roughly chopped
seeds from ½ pomegranate

for the mint yoghurt dressing:
80g yoghurt
a pinch of Himalayan pink salt
zest of ½ lemon
10g mint, chopped
a pinch of ground cinnamon

Melt 1 teaspoon of the coconut oil in a pan and add the garlic, fennel seeds and halloumi. Spread the halloumi around the pan so that it is covered in the garlic and fennel seeds and cook for about 1 minute on each side, until the halloumi is golden brown. Remove from the pan and set aside.

Keep the pan on the heat and add another teaspoon of the coconut oil. Chop the bottom off the baby gem lettuces and cut each bulb into quarters. Add these to the pan and gently sauté for about 1½–2 minutes until the leaves just begin to wilt. Transfer to a plate or serving bowl.

Bring a pan of water to the boil and add the salt. Once boiling, add the green beans and blanch for 2–3 minutes until just soft, then drain. If you have any precooked beans, you can throw them into the pan at the same time as the lettuce just to warm them up.

Chop the beans at an angle and toss through the lettuce with the mint and pomegranate. Return the halloumi to the pan.

Finally, make the yoghurt dressing by stirring all of the ingredients together in a glass or jug. Pour over the salad and serve.

>

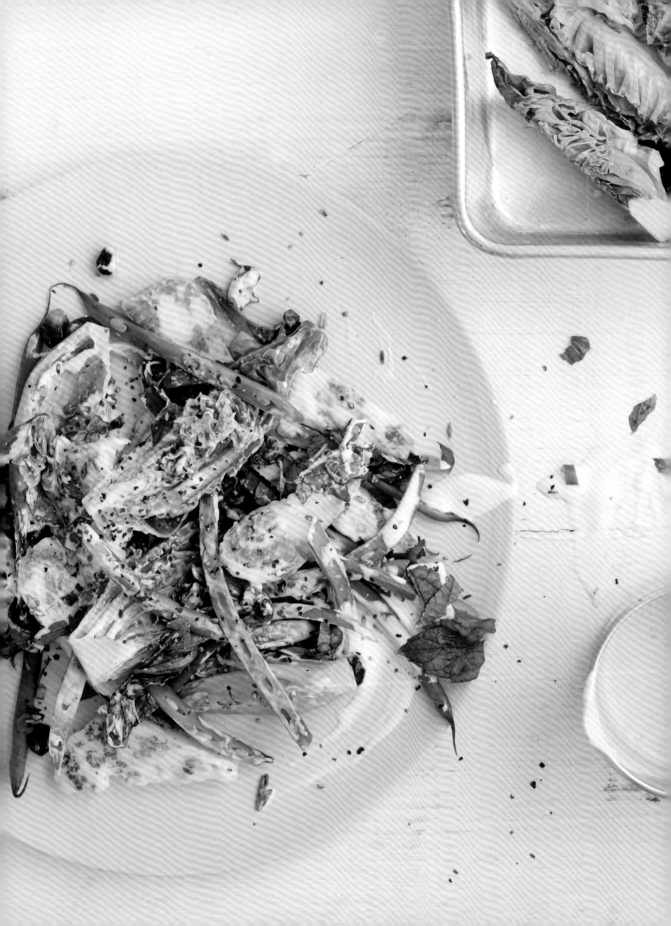

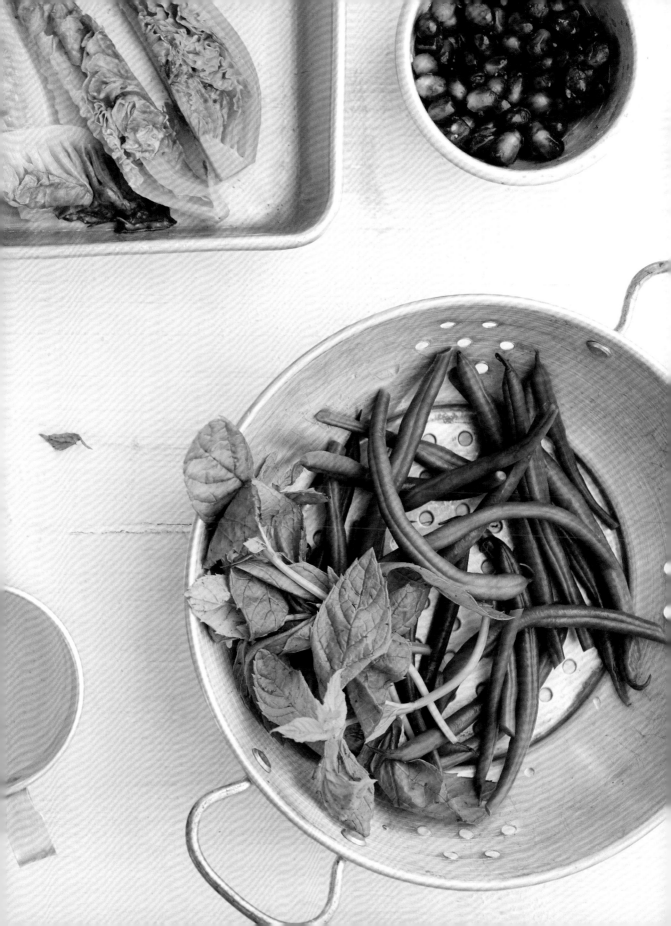

This is a great prep night dish. If you have some pre-blanched
broccoli and cooked noodles, you can pull this together
very quickly – just leave out the roasting of the broccoli and use
it blanched instead. All you need to do is soak some seaweed
for a couple of minutes and make the dressing.

SERVES 2

asian noodle salad

Preheat the oven to 180°C/160°C fan/gas mark 4.

Cook the soba noodles according to the packet instructions.
One minute before they are ready, add the edamame beans.
Bring to the boil again, then drain and pour some fresh boiling
water over them to get rid of the starch. Transfer to a bowl and
set aside.

Put the broccoli onto a baking tray, sprinkle with the sunflower
oil, salt and rice vinegar and put into the oven for 10 minutes
until just soft.

Soak the seaweed in cold water for about 5 minutes. Drain and
add to the soba noodles along with the herbs.

Combine all of the ingredients for the dressing in a glass or jug
and mix until thoroughly combined. Pour three-quarters of the
dressing over the noodles mixture and stir through.

Transfer to a serving plate or bowl and top with the broccoli,
sesame seeds, chopped chilli and spring onion. Drizzle over the
remaining dressing and serve.

100g soba (buckwheat)
   noodles
80g edamame beans
125g Tenderstem broccoli
1 tbsp sunflower oil
a pinch of Himalayan pink salt
¼ tsp brown rice vinegar
10g arame seaweed
5g mint leaves
4g coriander leaves
1 tbsp sesame seeds
2–3cm red chilli, finely
   chopped
1 spring onion, finely chopped

*for the ginger and lime
dressing:*
1cm piece of root ginger,
   grated
1 tbsp olive oil
1 tbsp sesame oil
1 tbsp brown rice vinegar
juice of 1 lime
1 tsp mirin
a pinch of Himalayan pink salt

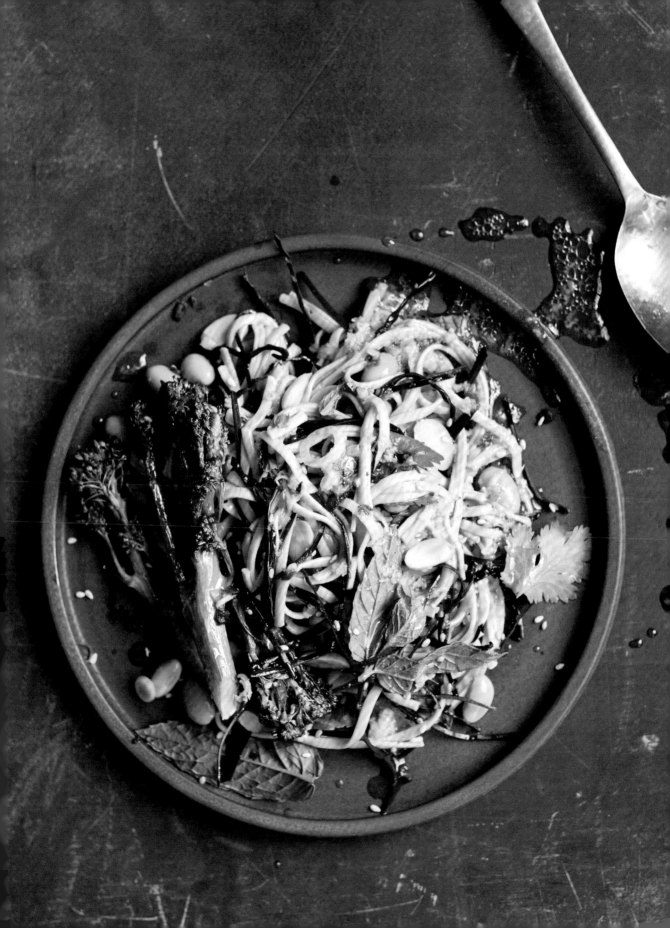

This is a quick and simple recipe that I first made at my office. It's a very versatile recipe. You could even try the blistering method with the courgette and pour the dressing over the top. I like to make up a big batch of this dressing and leave it in my fridge. It's so deliciously creamy and makes a tasty protein kick that transforms pretty much any salad or grain dish.

SERVES 1

blistered aubergine *and* courgette

Put the whole aubergine under the grill for 20 minutes, turning so that it blisters and chars on all sides.

In a frying pan, add the coconut oil and garlic and cook over a medium heat. After about 30 seconds, add the slices of courgette and cook for about 2–3 minutes on each side until they go golden brown.

Take off the heat and make the dressing.

Put the lemon juice, tahini, 4 tablespoons water and a pinch of salt into a blender and blitz until the mixture has a creamy smooth texture.

Holding the hot aubergine with a cloth, scrape the burnt skin off and into a bin. Once it is all off, put the aubergine onto a plate and scatter the courgette over the top.

Pour the dressing over and sprinkle with the black pepper, dill and lemon zest.

1 aubergine
1 tbsp coconut oil
2 cloves garlic, finely sliced
1 courgette (about 180g), sliced into 5mm rounds

for the dressing:
juice and zest of 1 lemon
4 tbsp tahini
a generous pinch of Himalayan pink salt
a sprinkling of freshly ground black pepper
10g dill, roughly chopped

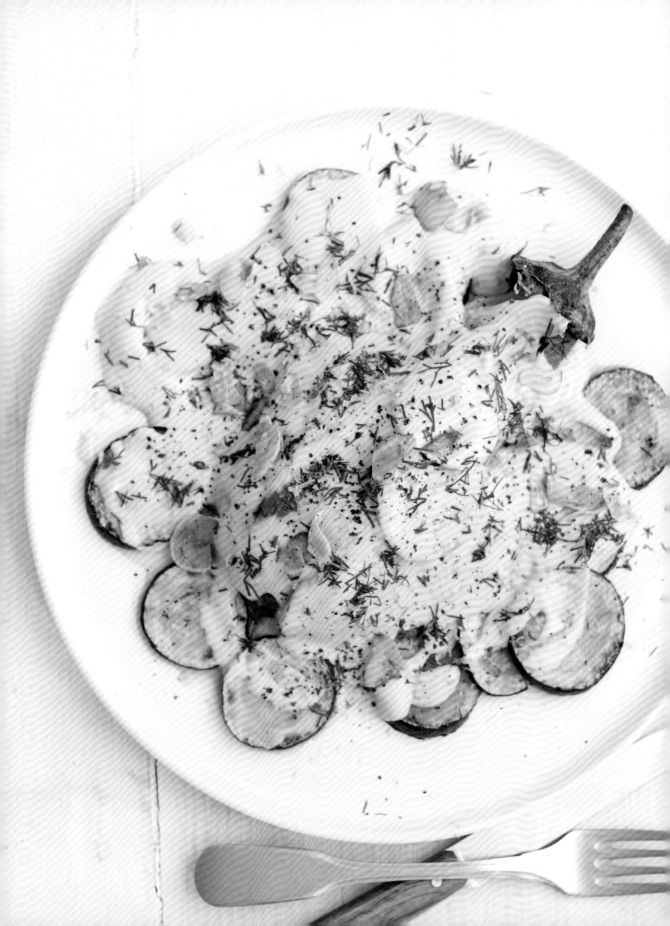

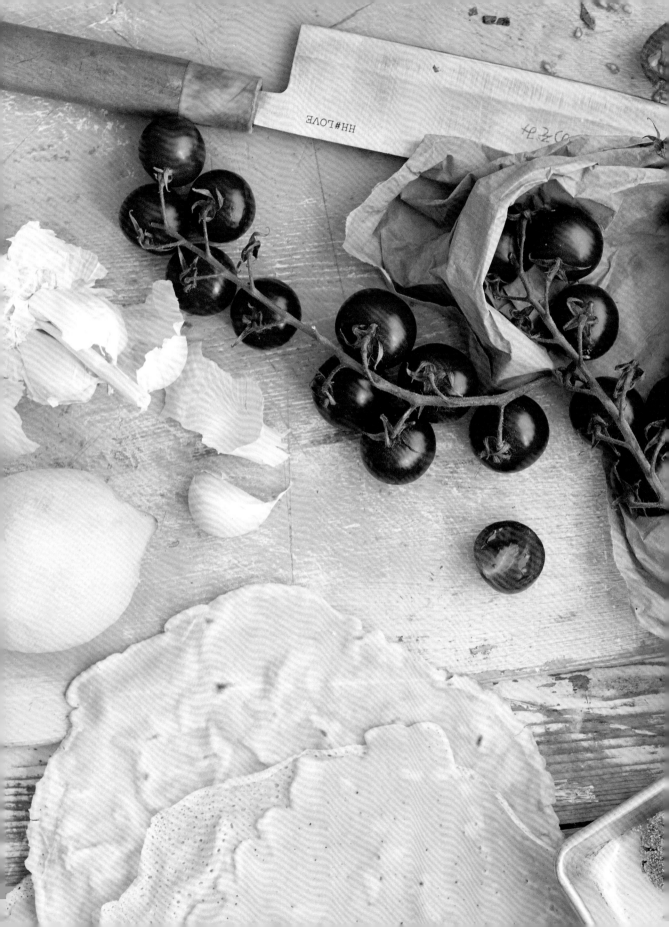

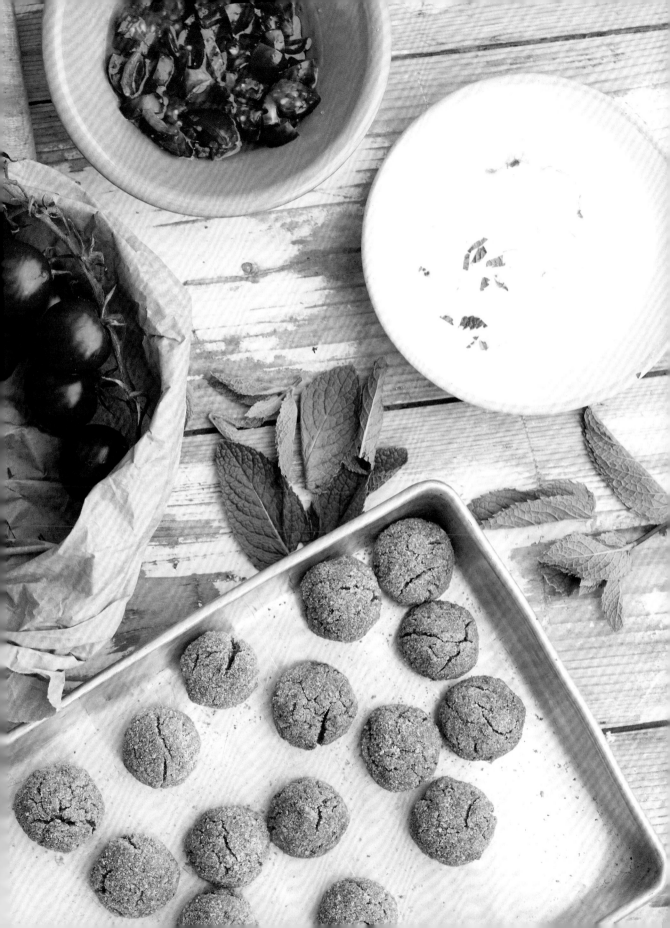

If you have already roasted the sweet potato and it's in your fridge, this is a great dish to whip together quickly. The falafels will keep in the fridge for about 3–4 days, so are great for taking to work for lunch. You could also try these with roasted beetroot or butternut squash.

MAKES 16 FALAFELS

sweet potato falafels

Preheat the oven to 180°C/160°C fan/gas mark 4.

Scoop out the flesh of the cooled roasted sweet potato into a food processor.

Grate the garlic into the processor and add the paprika, salt and sunflower oil and pulse until smooth. Add the coriander and pulse again. Stir in the quinoa flour.

Divide the mixture into 16 equal pieces and roll into balls. It is a wet mixture, but don't worry: roll them in the polenta and they will hold their shape perfectly. Bake in the oven for 25 minutes until crisp on the outside.

Combine the ingredients for the yoghurt dip and the tomato salsa in separate bowls. Serve the falafels with a mixed leaf salad and a gluten-free wrap, adding some dressing and salsa. You can use the taco recipe on page 98 but without baking them.

340g roasted sweet potato (500g raw sweet potato, roasted whole) (see page 12)
½ clove garlic, grated
¼ tsp smoked paprika
a pinch of Himalayan pink salt
½ tsp sunflower oil
20g coriander, roughly chopped
25g quinoa flour
polenta, for dusting

for the yoghurt dip:
180g goats' milk or dairy-free yoghurt
¼ clove garlic, grated
zest of 1 lemon
10g mint, chopped
a pinch of Himalayan pink salt

for the tomato salsa:
180g baby tomatoes, sliced
1 tbsp olive oil
a pinch of Himalayan pink salt

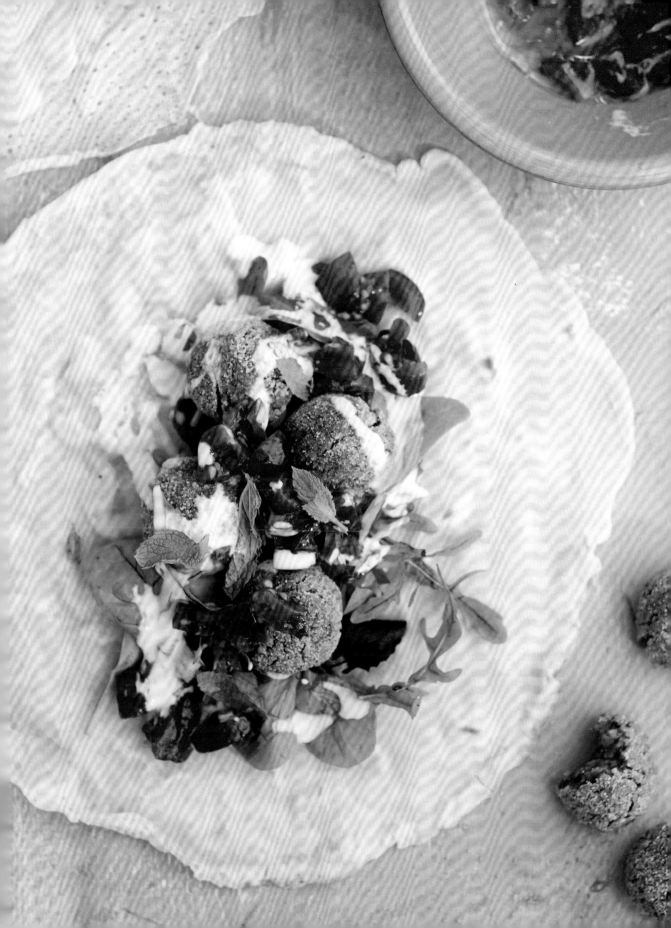

Here's a great technique to use with all your leftovers.
This version is a wonderful Asian-inspired sandwich, but I
have also eaten the nori sandwich with my roasted veg, some
rocket and a tahini dressing, which will also blow your mind!

SERVES 2

open nori sandwich
with sweet potato butter

Preheat the oven to 190°C/170°C fan/gas mark 5.

Fold the nori sheets in half. Brush a little water inside, then stick them together.

Put them on a baking sheet and place in the oven for 5 minutes to crisp up.

Scoop the sweet potato flesh into a bowl and beat with the coconut oil until it's smooth. Set aside while you make the salad.

Combine the dressing ingredients with 1 tablespoon water and mix well. Put the radishes, salad leaves, cucumber, sprouts (if using) and spring onion into a bowl, add the dressing and toss well.

When the nori comes out of the oven, spread each crisp doubled sheet with the sweet potato butter and pile the salad on the top.

4 sheets of nori seaweed

80g roasted sweet potato (120g raw sweet potato, roasted whole) (see page 12)

1 tsp coconut oil, at room temperature

3 radishes (50g), thinly sliced

10g wild salad or rocket leaves

150g cucumber, spiralised (see page 74)

5g radish or alfalfa sprouts (optional)

1 spring onion, thinly sliced

for the miso dressing:

1 tbsp sweet miso

½ tsp sesame oil

zest of ½ lime

a pinch of Himalayan pink salt

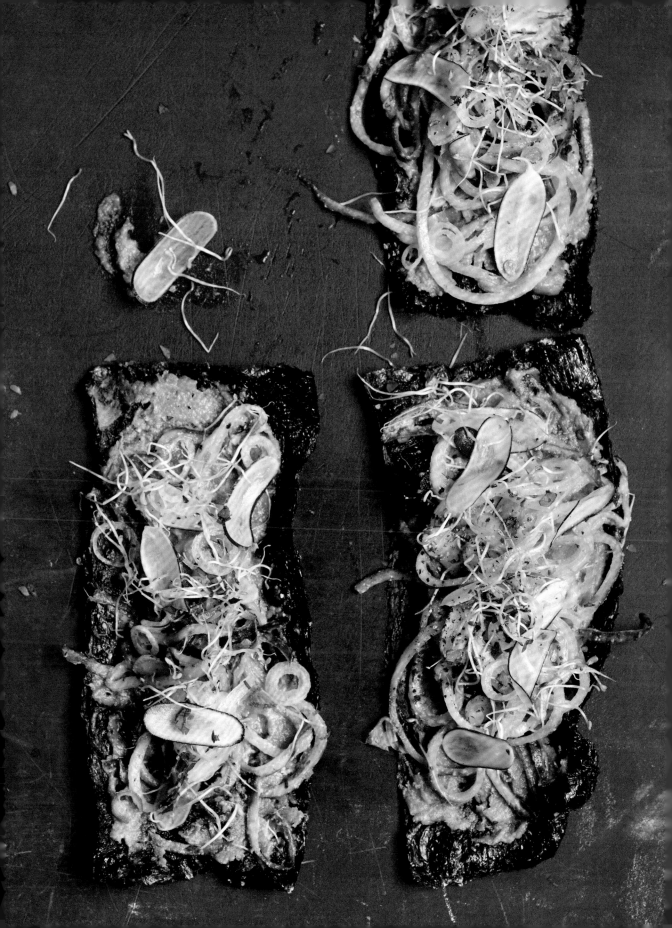

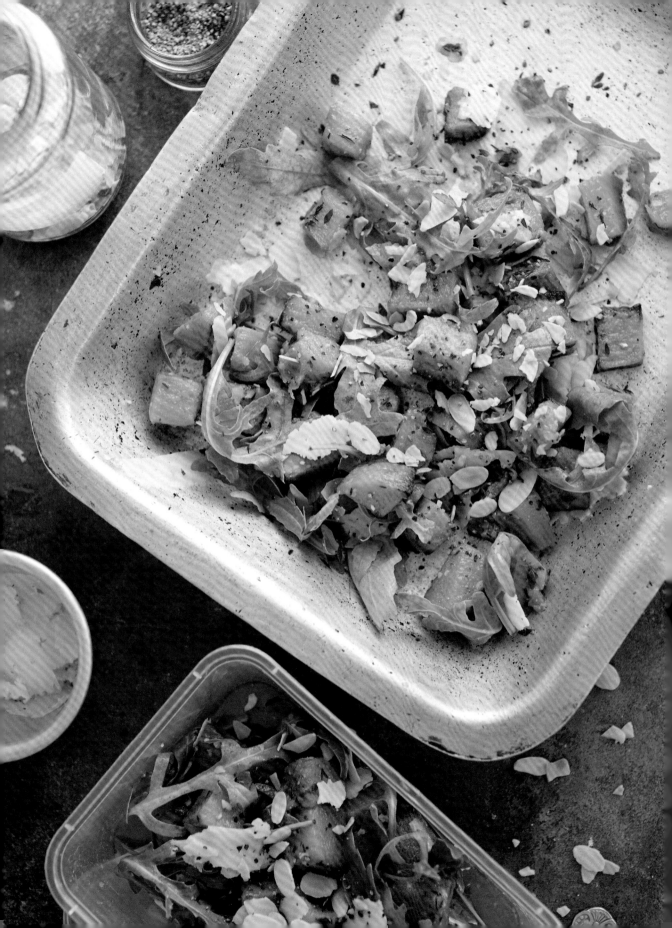

This really is such a quick and completely rewarding salad.
The combination of thyme, cumin and manchego in this salad is just
one of the best. If you can't find manchego, pecorino would work
really well too. The salad is great with warm or cold butternut squash
– both are just as comforting and delicious!

SERVES 2

butternut squash *and* thyme salad

440g roasted butternut squash (600g raw butternut squash, peeled and chopped into 1cm cubes) (see page 12)

10g thyme leaves, roughly chopped

a pinch of Himalayan pink salt

a generous pinch of freshly ground black pepper

1 tbsp walnut oil

a pinch of ground cumin

35g manchego cheese

60g rocket

10g flaked almonds

Put the butternut squash into a bowl with the thyme leaves, salt, pepper, walnut oil and cumin and gently combine with your hands until the squash is evenly coated.

Next, slice the manchego cheese using a potato peeler or mandoline to get really nice, thin slices. Stir them through the squash.

Place the rocket on a plate and spoon the butternut mixture on top. Sprinkle with flaked almonds and serve.

1+2 ›

I first made this recipe with some of the sweetest, most delicious cherry tomatoes and the flavour was literally incredible. I always try to buy tomatoes on the vine, the reddest bunch I can find – they are usually the best flavour-wise. I am also a sucker for eggs on a Sunday night, and this is one of the most comforting dishes out there. There are three ways that you can do this recipe – either with sliced, grated or precooked potatoes.

SERVES 2

sweet potato baked eggs

Preheat the oven to 180°C/160°C fan/gas mark 4.

Finely slice the sweet potato – each slice should be around 2mm thick. Use a mandoline to do this if you have one. The thinner you slice the sweet potatoes, the quicker the cooking time.

Line 1 or 2 small ovenproof casserole or pie dishes with the sweet potatoes.

Next, put the tomatoes, garlic, walnut oil and salt into a food processor and blitz until roughly chopped – the tomatoes should have roughly quartered in size.

Pour the tomato mixture over the sweet potatoes and bake in the oven for 30–35 minutes.

When they are almost soft, stir in the tarragon (if using), and crack the eggs over the top. Bake in the oven for a further 6–8 minutes, or until the whites are no longer translucent. Serve straight away with a sprinkling of black pepper over the top.

150g raw sweet potato, peeled
230g cherry tomatoes
1 clove garlic, grated
1 tbsp walnut or olive oil
a generous pinch of Himalayan pink salt
10g tarragon, roughly chopped (optional)
2 eggs
a pinch of freshly ground black pepper

>>●

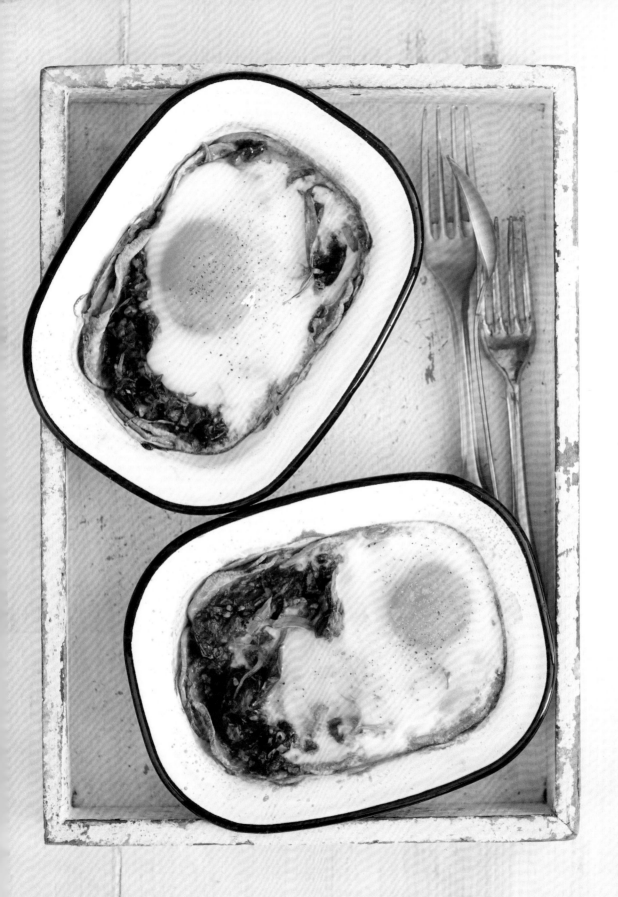

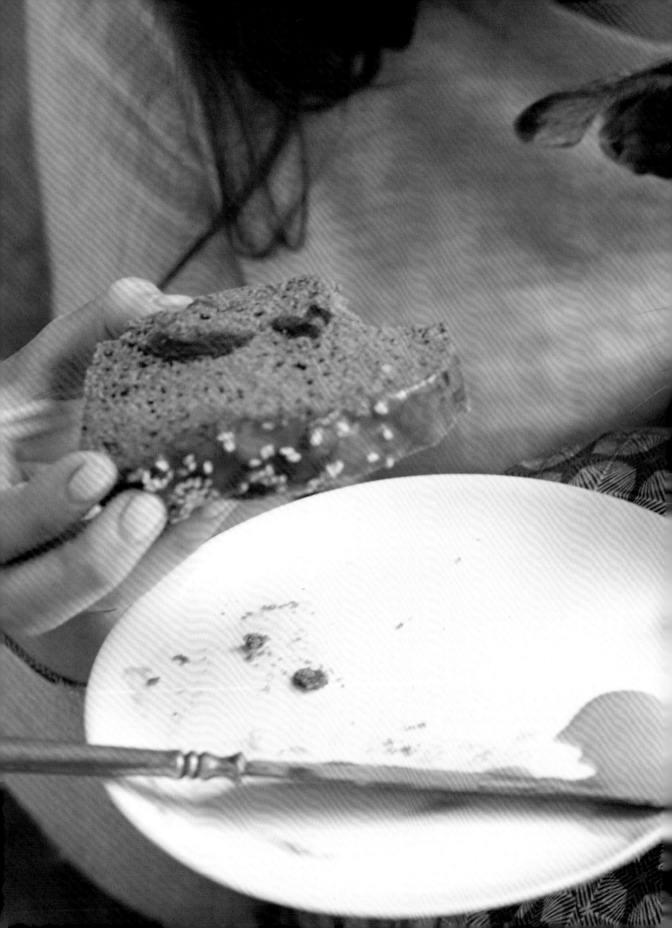

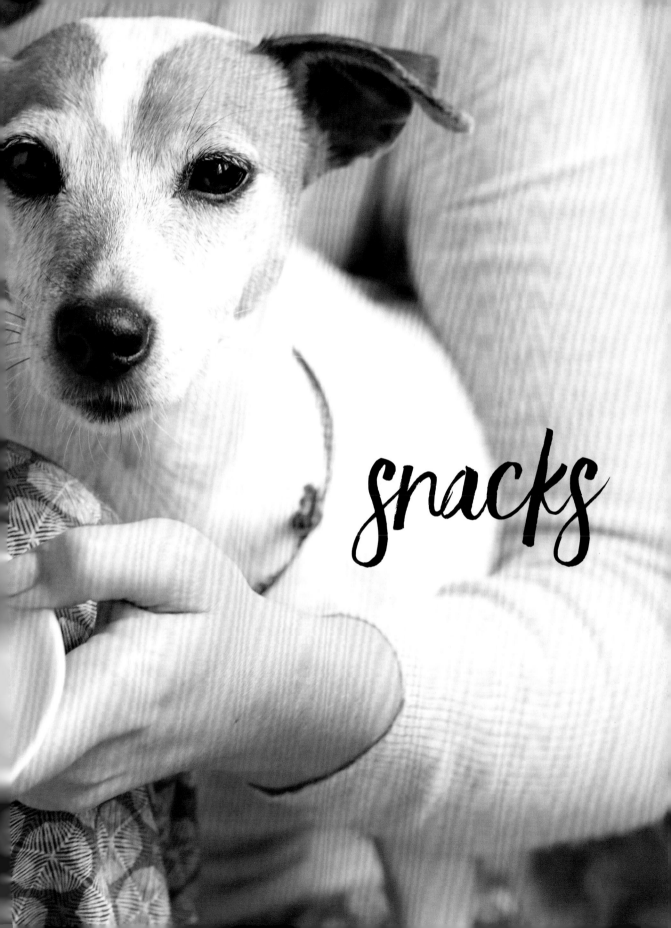

snacks

Bruschette remind me of being on holiday in the
summer in Europe. Here I have added a few new tweaks to
make them a little more zesty and interesting.

SERVES 3

bruschette three ways

Take three slices of the soda bread and generously brush both
sides with the olive oil. Heat a griddle pan until hot, then
griddle each slice on both sides until nicely charred. Top each
slice with one or all of the below options.

For the tapenade topping, place all of the ingredients in a
blender and gently pulse to a rough paste. Taste and add a
little more salt or lemon juice if needed. Spread on the
bruschette and garnish with sprigs of watercress.

For the tomato and broad bean topping, preheat the oven to
180°C/160°C fan/gas mark 4. Roughly chop the tomatoes and
place on a baking tray lined with baking parchment. Sprinkle
with the garlic, a pinch of salt and 1 tablespoon of the olive oil
and roast in the oven for 10–12 minutes until soft.

Place the broad beans in a saucepan, cover with water and
bring to the boil. Add the peas, bring back to the boil, then
drain and cool under the cold tap.

Transfer three-quarters of the pea and bean mixture to a
blender, add the remaining olive oil and the lemon juice and
blitz to a rough texture. Scrape into a bowl and stir through the
remaining peas and beans, the mint, dill and salt and pepper.
Taste and add more lemon juice or salt if needs be.

Spread the broad bean dip evenly over the bruschette and
spoon the roasted tomatoes on top.

For the goats' cheese and radish topping, spread the cheese
evenly over the toasted bread. Put all the remaining ingredients
into a bowl, reserving a little of the lime zest, and toss well.
Carefully pile the radishes over the goats' cheese and sprinkle
the top with black pepper and the extra lime zest.

Soda bread (see page 46)
1½ tbsp olive oil

for the tapenade topping:
170g olives, pitted
1 tbsp olive oil
½ tsp apple cider vinegar
5g parsley
juice of ½ lemon
5g basil
¼ clove garlic
watercress, to garnish
Himalayan pink salt

*for the tomato, broad bean
and mint topping:*
2 large tomatoes
1 clove garlic, roughly chopped
2½ tbsp olive oil
180g broad beans
75g peas
juice of ½ large lemon
15g mint, roughly chopped
5g dill, roughly chopped
freshly ground black pepper
Himalayan pink salt

*for the goats' cheese and
radish topping:*
soft goats' cheese
3 radishes, finely sliced
zest and juice of ¼ lime
2–3 large mint leaves, roughly
    chopped
3–4 drops of brown rice or
    apple cider vinegar

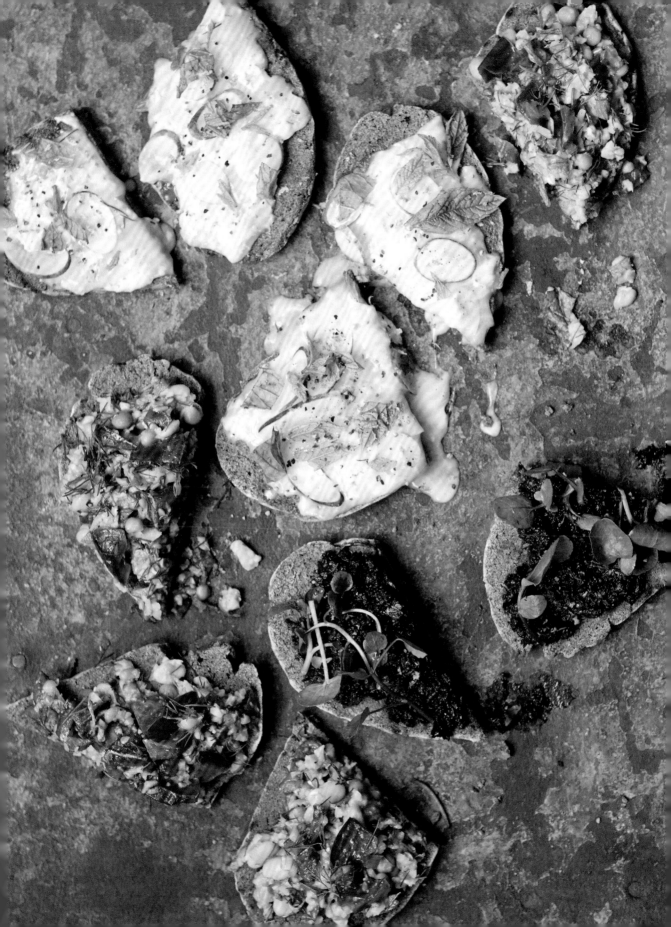

This loaf is a fruit loaf with a twist, being full of wonderful dates and fragrant cardamom. It is quick to bring together and ideal for enjoying warm with a hot cup of tea. You can also toast it and spread with coconut oil for an even more delicious treat.

SERVES 8

date, cardamom AND tahini loaf

Preheat the oven to 150°C/130°C fan/gas mark 2. Line a 23 × 13cm loaf tin with baking parchment.

Crush the cardamom pods in a mortar, discarding the husks.

Put the flours into a bowl with the bicarbonate of soda, baking powder, salt and xanthan gum, add the cardamom seeds and mix together.

Beat the eggs in a separate bowl, then stir in the milk, syrup, tahini and sunflower oil. Mix well, then stir in the chopped dates.

Gradually add the flour mixture to the wet mixture, stirring until well combined. It is meant to be thick.

Scrape the batter into the prepared tin and make sure the top is even.

Bake in the oven for 40–45 minutes until a knife inserted in the centre comes out clean. Turn out of the tin and leave to cool.

To make the icing, mix the tahini and syrup together in a bowl with 2 tablespoons water and drizzle over the top of the loaf. Sprinkle with the sesame seeds.

6 cardamom pods
160g gluten-free plain flour
80g teff flour
1 tsp bicarbonate of soda
1½ tsp baking powder
½ tsp Himalayan pink salt
1 tsp xanthan gum
2 eggs
125ml dairy-free milk
100ml coconut blossom or
   date syrup
50ml tahini
50ml sunflower or coconut oil
180g dates, chopped
1 tsp sesame seeds, to garnish

for the icing:
35g tahini
20ml coconut blossom syrup

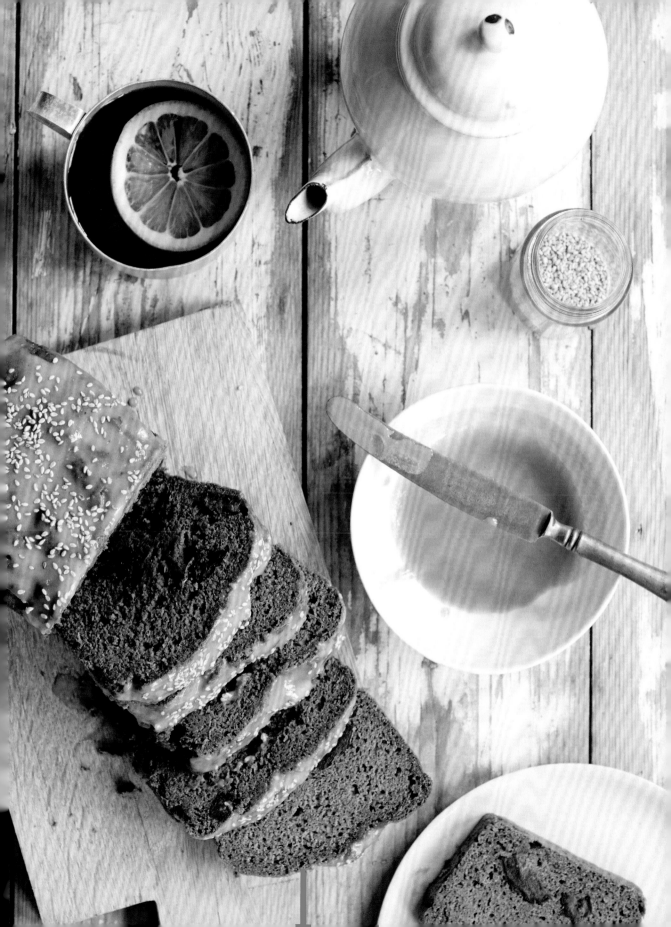

Coffee used to be a real weakness for my husband – we are
talking numerous cups a day. He now hardly touches the stuff, having
been introduced to Yannoh barley coffee. It tastes just the same,
but contains none of the caffeine. This is a really dreamy and
refreshing milkshake for a hot day – I just love those mocha flavours.
If you have just done a workout, try adding a tablespoon
of your protein powder too. If you are coeliac and cannot have
barley, you can use dandelion coffee instead.

SERVES 2

iced mocha milkshake

Put all of the ingredients into a high-speed blender with
185ml water and blitz until smooth and ice cold.

Pour into an ice-filled glass and enjoy.

250ml almond milk (bought or
see page 52)
1 large banana (about 120g),
peeled
1 tbsp cashew or almond
butter
¼ tsp vanilla extract
3 whole dates, pitted
pinch of Himalayan pink salt
1 tbsp instant barley coffee
1 tbsp raw cacao powder
large handful of ice

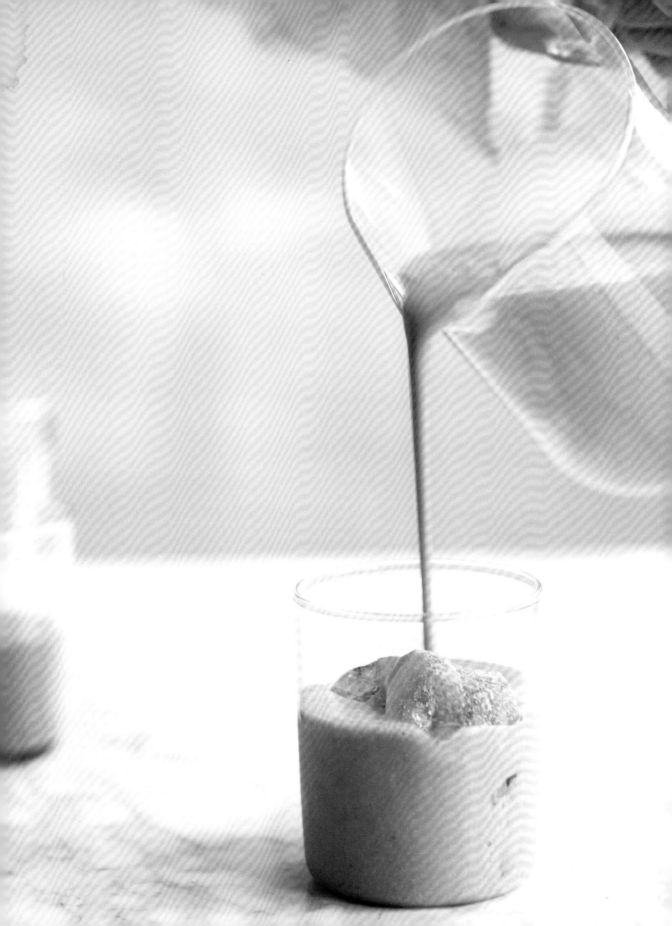

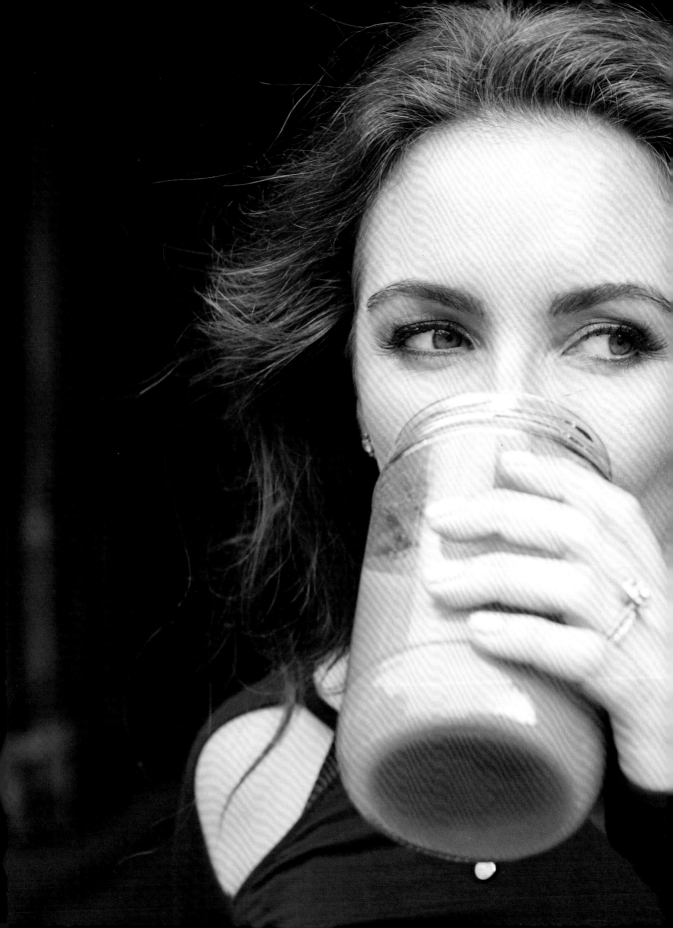

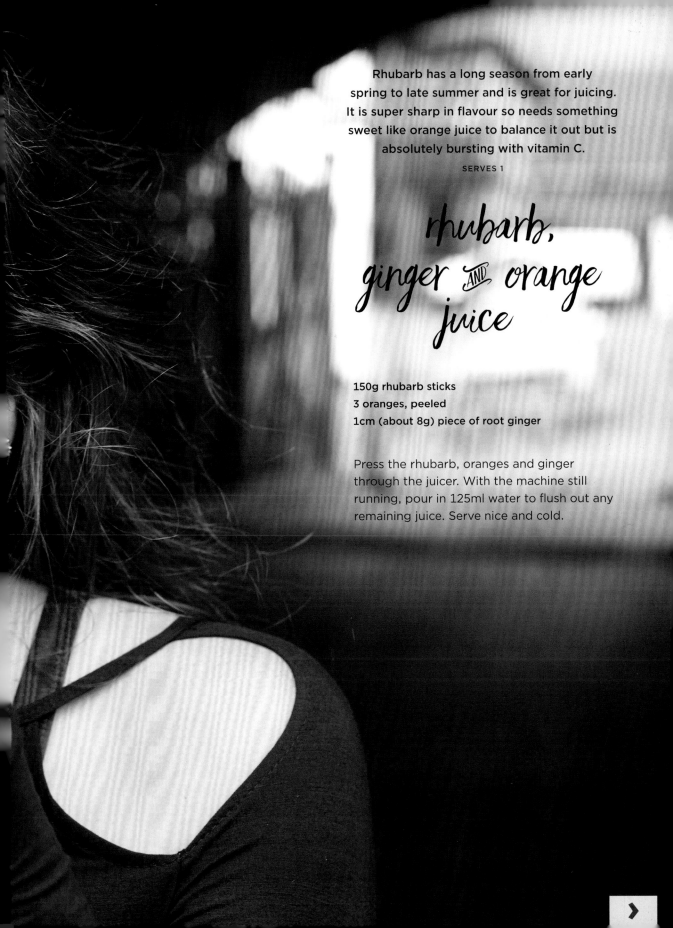

Rhubarb has a long season from early spring to late summer and is great for juicing. It is super sharp in flavour so needs something sweet like orange juice to balance it out but is absolutely bursting with vitamin C.

SERVES 1

rhubarb, ginger AND orange juice

150g rhubarb sticks
3 oranges, peeled
1cm (about 8g) piece of root ginger

Press the rhubarb, oranges and ginger through the juicer. With the machine still running, pour in 125ml water to flush out any remaining juice. Serve nice and cold.

You will see from how much avocado I use in this book and all my books that I love to eat it. I get asked all the time what is the one ingredient I can't live without and I always mention this green fruit. Its nutritional properties are amazing, being full of vitamin E that is great for the skin, and also full of essential fats. It is so creamy you can use it in anything from dips and soups to smoothies and desserts. Also, it is really alkaline, which is the best news ever!

SERVES 2

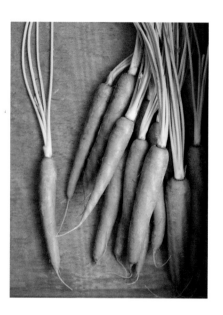

avocado AND tahini dip

Put all ingredients into a blender or food processor and blend until smooth.

Serve with crackers or crudités.

2 avocados
1 small clove garlic
juice of ½ lemon
2 tbsp tahini

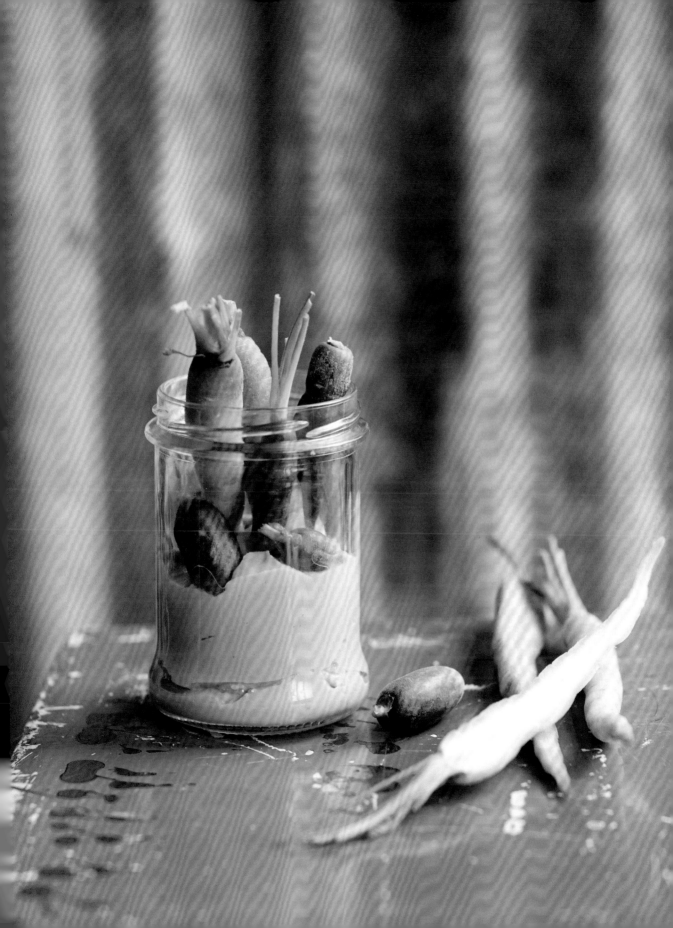

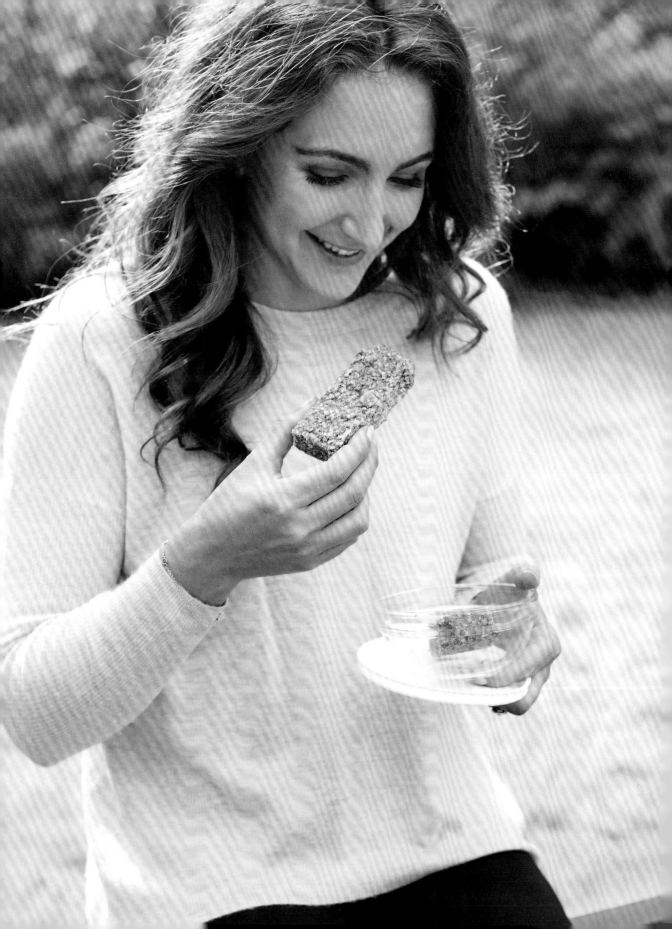

I love a good granola bar, and these little morsels of fun are not to be missed. They are packed with protein and very quick to make. You can also freeze them and pull them out as you need them. I love to make a big batch and then always have them on hand. They will keep in an airtight container in the fridge for about 10 days.

MAKES 10 BARS

quinoa granola bars

200g dates, stones removed

4 tbsp almond butter

125g quinoa flakes

30g flaked almonds, plus extra to garnish (optional)

zest of 1 lemon

10g poppy or sesame seeds

If you can't find quinoa flakes, use oats. And why not try with orange zest instead of lemon, or cashew butter instead of almond?

Preheat the oven to 170°C/150°C fan/gas mark 3 and line a baking tray with baking parchment.

Put the dates, 60ml water and the almond butter into a food processor and blend until it forms a thick, sticky paste. Stir in the quinoa flakes, almonds, lemon zest and poppy or sesame seeds until well mixed.

Spread the mixture out in your lined baking tray so it is about 2cm thick. Garnish with extra flaked almonds, if using.

Put into the oven for 10 minutes, then transfer to a wire rack to cool before tucking in with a cup of tea.

These nori chips are my new obsession instead of crisps.
They are so quick to make, and really tasty with the salsa, and
also with the Creamy cauliflower and tahini dip (see
page 184) or the broad bean and mint topping from the
Bruschette three ways recipe (see page 158).

SERVES 2

nori chips
with cucumber salsa

Preheat the oven to 180°C/160°C fan/gas mark 4.

Cut the nori sheets in half and brush one side of each piece
with water so that it is evenly coated but not too wet. Press
each wet half onto a dry half.

Cut each double nori sheet into triangles and sprinkle each side
with salt and pepper. Place on a baking sheet and bake in the
oven for 5 minutes until nice and crispy.

To prepare the salsa, put the cucumber into a bowl with the
remaining ingredients. Stir well.

Spoon the salsa onto the crisps and enjoy.

3 sheets of nori seaweed
a generous pinch of
    Himalayan pink salt
a generous pinch of freshly
    ground black pepper

for the cucumber salsa:
200g cucumber, finely diced
2 spring onions, finely diced
2 tsp brown rice vinegar
2 tsp sesame oil
1 tbsp olive oil
1cm piece of root ginger,
    grated
a generous pinch of
    Himalayan pink salt
zest of ¼ lime
juice of ½ lime
a generous pinch of freshly
    ground black pepper
5g coriander, roughly
    chopped
½ tsp tamari

❯

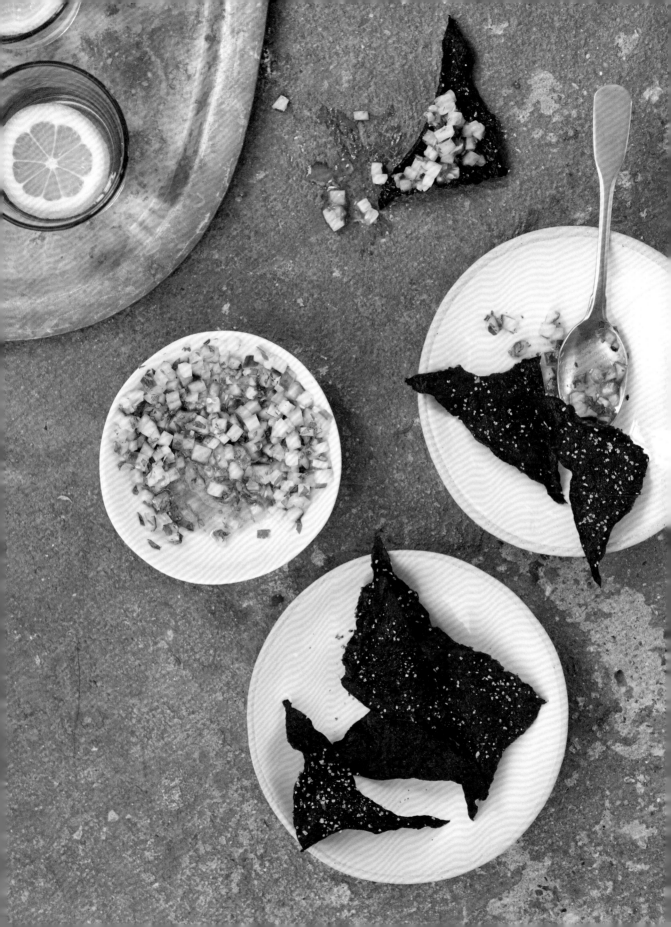

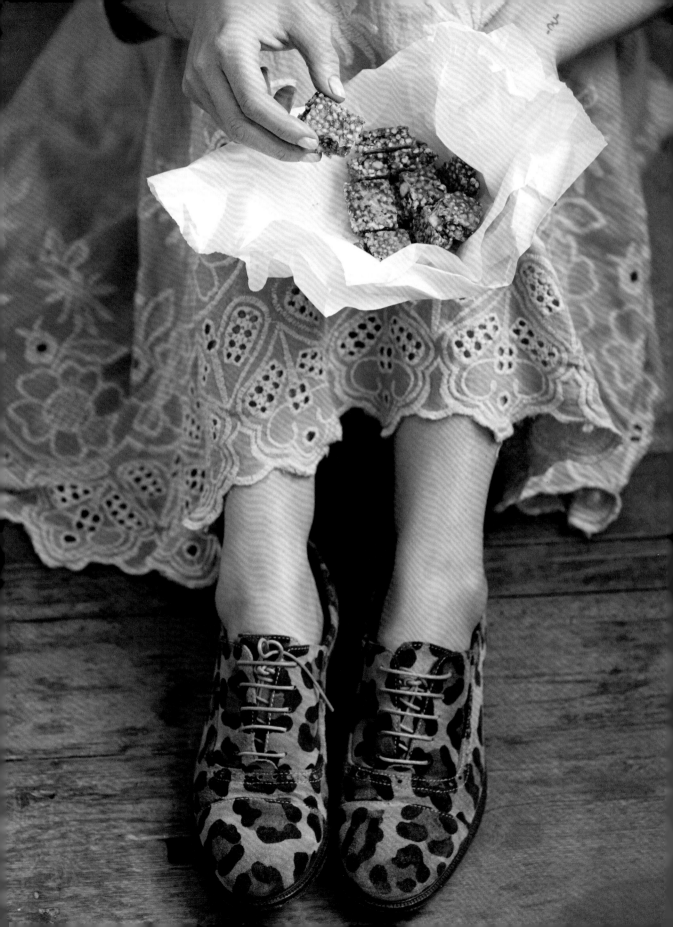

These are so delicious and perfect for a sweet treat. I like to keep them in the fridge or freezer for a rainy day so that I always have something to enjoy if I get a sweet craving.

MAKES 12–15 BITES

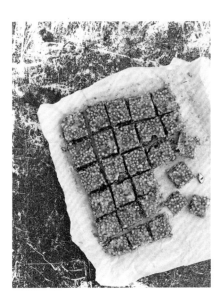

puffed quinoa *AND* buckwheat granola bites

140g dates, stones removed

85g coconut oil, at room temperature

1 tbsp date syrup

¼ tsp vanilla extract

20g puffed quinoa

40g whole buckwheat groats

50g shelled pistachios

a generous pinch of Himalayan pink salt

Put the dates, coconut oil, date syrup and vanilla extract into a blender and blitz until it forms a nice thick paste – the mixture may separate, but don't worry about this.

Transfer the mixture to a bowl and add the remaining ingredients. Stir until really well combined.

Line a 20 × 30cm baking tray with baking parchment and press the mixture into it so it is about 3cm thick – it will hold its shape, so don't worry if it doesn't fill the tray.

Put into the fridge to set for 1–2 hours. Remove from the fridge and cut into little bite-sized cubes. Store in an airtight container for up to 2 weeks, or a month in the freezer.

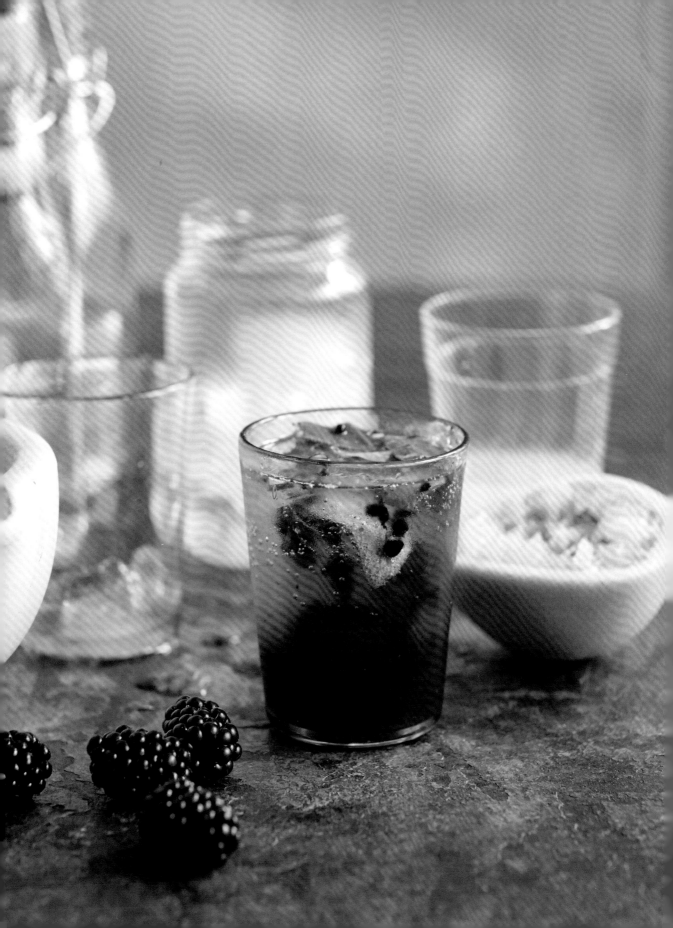

This is possibly one of the most refreshing drinks ever and is a complete showstopper if you serve it to anyone on soft drinks at a dinner party. Blackberries and sage are the perfect partners, so drink up!

SERVES 1

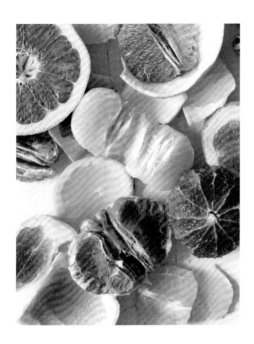

blackberry *AND* sage spritzer

50g blackberries

2 tbsp fresh grapefruit juice

1 sage leaf, plus extra to garnish

90g crushed ice

250ml soda water

In a small bowl, crush together the blackberries with the grapefruit juice and sage leaf. Put the crushed ice into a glass, pour the blackberry mixture over the top and fill to the top with the soda water. Serve straight away, garnished with a few additional sage leaves.

Kids love these because they are crunchy and naturally sweet, so they make a great healthy snack to give them that sweet kick. Oh, and big kids like them too!

SERVES 2–3 AS A SNACK

apple *AND* rosemary crisps

Preheat the oven to its lowest temperature.

Remove the apple stalks then slice each fruit into rounds about 2–3mm thick.

Break the rosemary into pieces and place into a bowl with the apple slices and lemon. Toss together gently with your hands and then transfer to a baking tray, laying everything out flat.

Bake in the oven for 2 hours until the apple slices are crispy.

2 eating apples
2 sprigs of rosemary
juice of ½ lemon

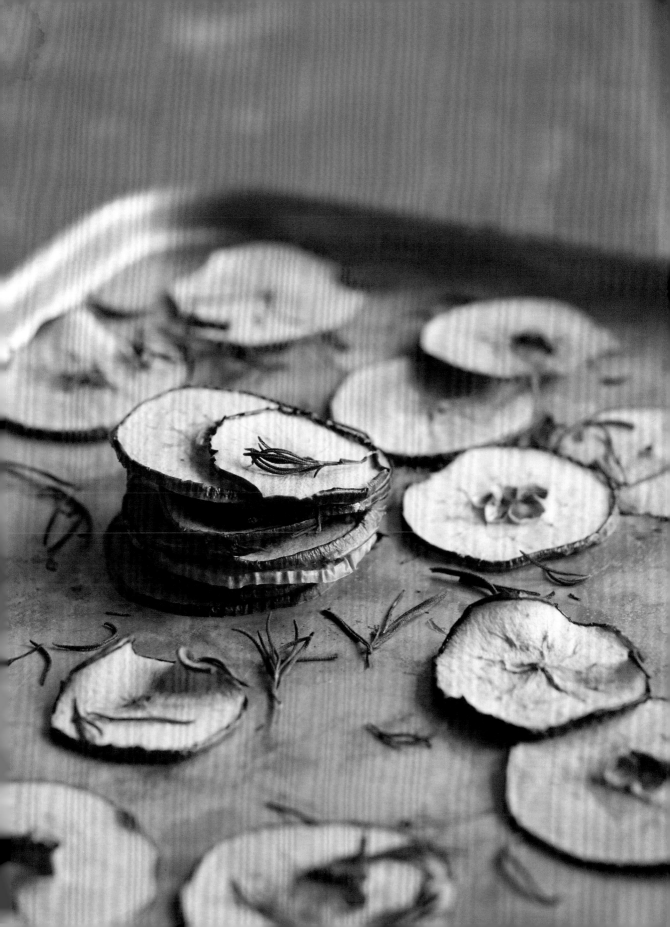

This is an insanely delicious remedy if you are feeling under the weather. The addition of baobab powder adds an extra potent dose of vitamin C and is also incredibly rehydrating for the body – both properties are vital when you have a cold or flu. A hot drink always seems to soothe the soul when you are feeling low or unwell, and the addition of aromatic star anise and cinnamon makes for a completely delicious, healthy soother. Add some grated ginger too if you would like a bit more of a kick to clear the sinuses.

SERVES 2

apple *and* baobab 'hot toddy'

Juice the apples and transfer the juice to a pan. Add the remaining ingredients and slowly bring to the boil. Allow to simmer for 3 minutes before turning off the heat and straining the juice.

juice of 3 apples (400ml)
3 star anise
3 slices of root ginger
a generous pinch of ground cinnamon
1 tsp baobab powder

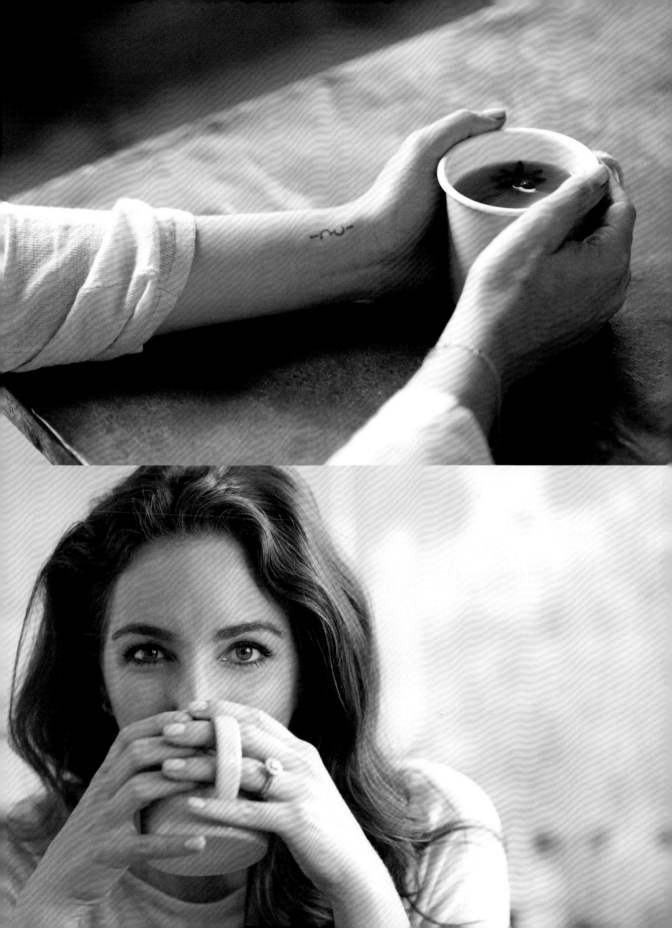

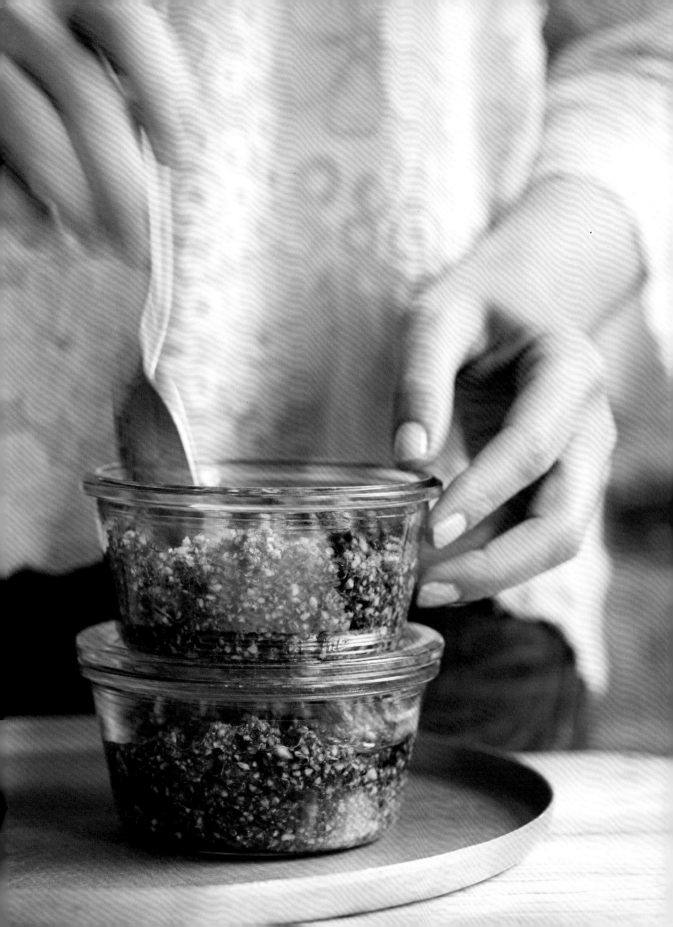

I love pesto and it's great to have a big amount tucked away in the freezer so you can make things like the Spring minestrone soup (see page 70), Buckwheat and pesto ravioli (see page 124) or just a simple pasta pesto dish. Also a great one for kids, you can change the nuts and herbs to suit your taste.

MAKES 350G PESTO (1 SMALL KILNER JAR)

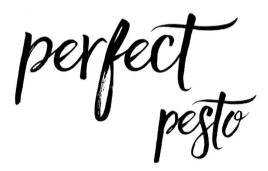

220g cashews

1 large clove garlic

40g parsley

20g coriander

¼ tsp onion seeds

125ml olive oil

a pinch of Himalayan pink salt

a pinch of freshly ground
   black pepper

Put the cashews, garlic, parsley, coriander and onion seeds in a food processor and process until the mixture is crumb-like. Add the olive oil, salt and pepper and pulse again.

Use straight away or put into ice-cube trays and freeze for a later date, just warming as you need it.

I don't think I have met anyone who doesn't like hummus, and this is a great quick and tasty one to make, especially if you have the pesto in the freezer. All you need to do is heat it up for 2 minutes with a splash of water before adding to the rest of the ingredients.

SERVES 2–3

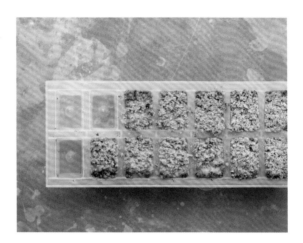

pesto hummus spread

Put all the ingredients into a food processor with 60ml water and blend until completely smooth and velvety. Enjoy as a side dish with salad or as a dip.

250g cooked chickpeas
50g Perfect pesto (see page 181)
juice of 1 lemon
1 tbsp oil
a pinch of Himalayan pink salt
¼ tsp ground cumin

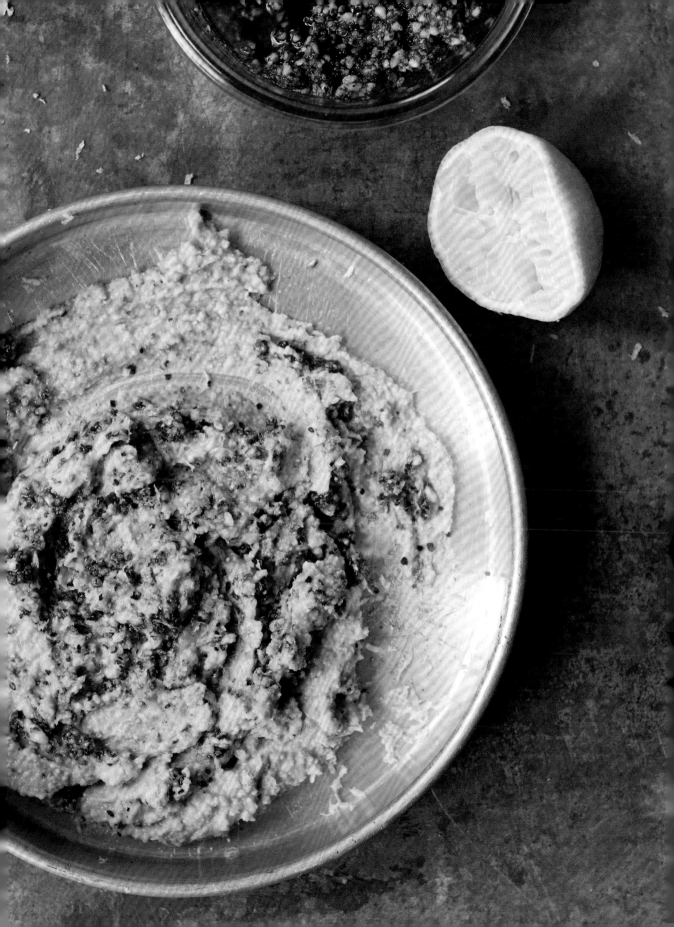

I wanted to create a different type of hummus and this is the result. I love how creamy cauliflower gets, and adding tahini gives a great protein kick to it. If you are roasting cauliflower just for this recipe, make double and add it to your salads – it's a great addition.

SERVES 2

creamy cauliflower *and* tahini dip

Put the roasted cauliflower into a food processor or blender with the tahini and lemon zest and blend until smooth. If you need more liquid, you can add 60ml water. Transfer to a serving bowl.

To make the spice scatter, toast the seeds in a dry frying pan for 2 minutes or until toasted and smelling aromatic. Remove from the heat and leave to cool slightly. Mix the sumac, lemon zest and parsley with the toasted seeds and scatter over the dip.

Serve the dip alongside a salad or as a traditional dip with crudités and crackers.

170g roasted cauliflower florets (260g raw cauliflower) (see page 12)
2 tbsp tahini
zest of 1 lemon

for the spice scatter:
½ tsp coriander seeds
½ tsp cumin seeds
½ tsp fennel seeds
1 tsp sesame seeds
½ tsp sumac
finely grated zest of ½ lemon
1 tbsp chopped parsley

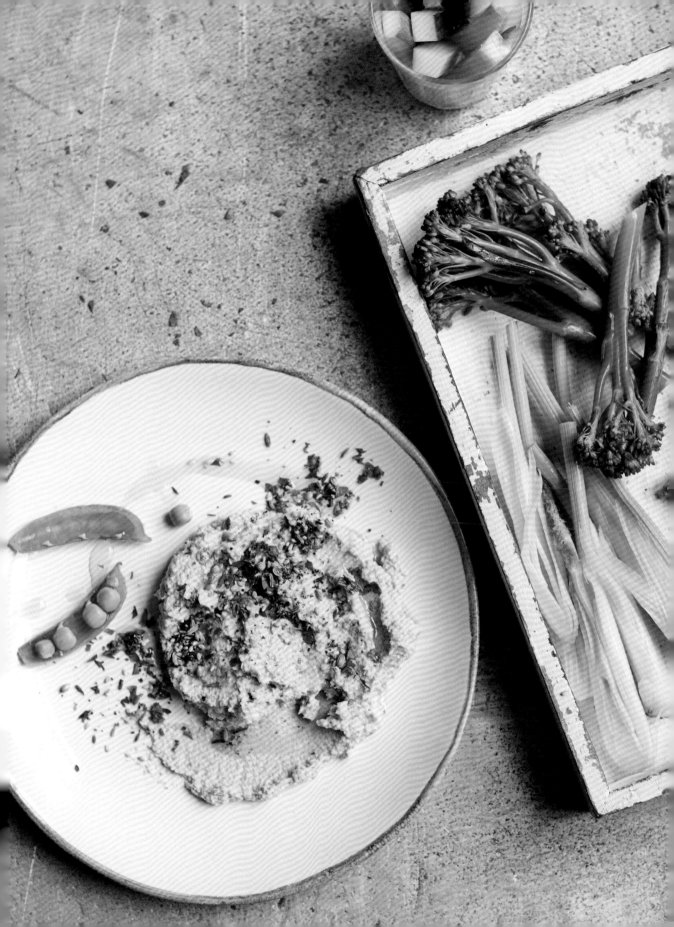

I hate leftovers, so when I make almond milk, I like to get inventive
with the pulp. My husband was craving biscuits so I made these for us
one rainy afternoon – they went down a little too well.

MAKES 15 BITES

almond pulp chewy bites

Preheat the oven to 200°C/180°C fan/gas mark 6.

Put the almond pulp, date syrup and vanilla extract into a bowl and mix in the flour. Add a little almond milk, if necessary, to loosen the mixture and make it less crumbly.

Divide the dough into 15 equal pieces. Roll them into balls and flatten a little. If you want to add the jam filling, press your thumb into the middle to make a little well. Try to smooth out any cracks, then put the circles onto a baking sheet and bake for 10 minutes.

If adding the jam, remove the bites from the oven and fill the little holes. Put back into the oven for a further 10 minutes. If you are not adding the jam, the bites will just need a further 5 minutes' cooking. Once golden brown on top, they should be ready.

Sprinkle a few sesame seeds over the jam topping if you wish. Leave the bites to cool and enjoy with a cup of tea.

175g almond pulp from the Almond milk, plus a dash of the milk itself (see page 52)
60g date syrup
½ tsp vanilla extract
55g gluten-free plain flour
Blueberry jam, for the filling (optional) (see page 56)
sesame seeds, to sprinkle (optional)

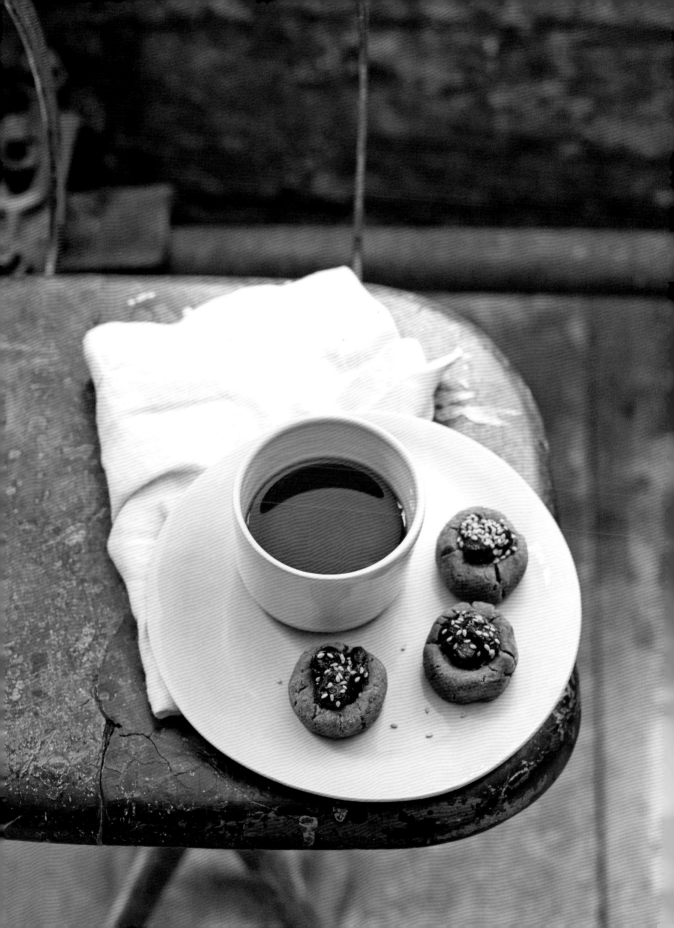

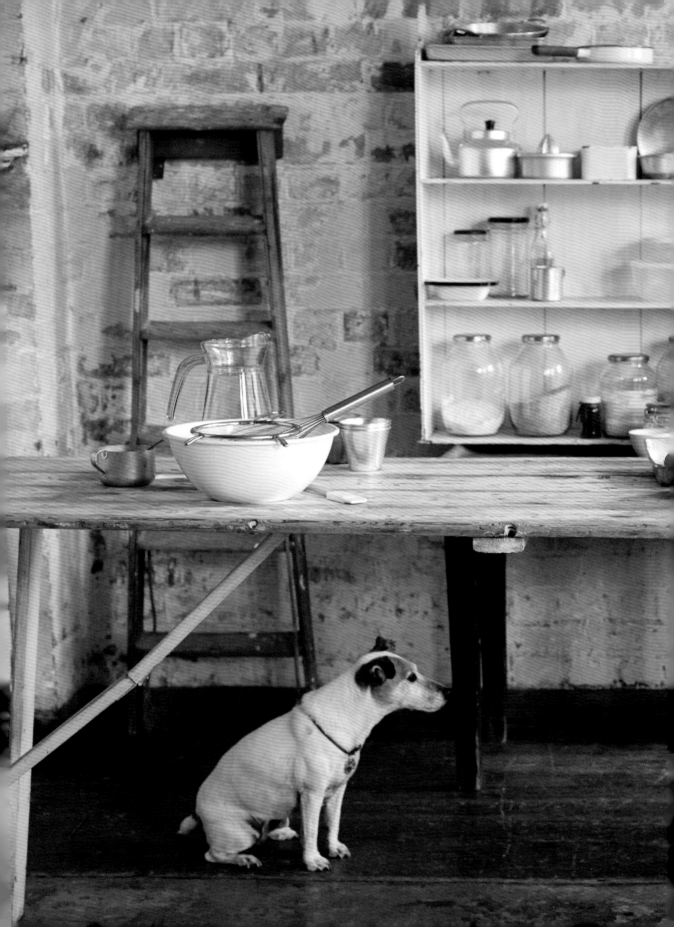

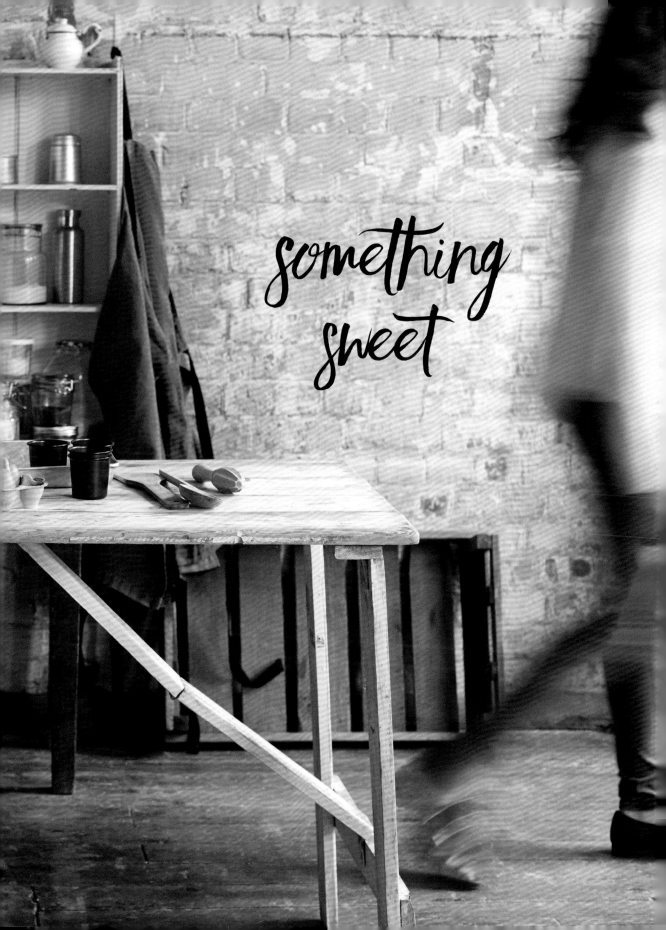

something
sweet

This gives you everything you need from a cake – it's moist
and sweet, delicious and satisfying. If you don't have peaches,
you could try it with pears in the winter months, or put a
banana down the centre of the cake. There are so many nice
variations you can try with this. It also looks gorgeous
when you slice it in half and see the fruit.

SERVES 6–8

peach *and* almond cake

Preheat the oven to 190°C/170°C fan/gas mark 5 and line a
24 × 14cm loaf tin with baking parchment.

Put the ground almonds into a bowl with the buckwheat flour,
baking powder, bicarbonate of soda and salt and combine.

In a separate bowl, whisk the eggs, then stir in the vanilla,
chopped peach, agave syrup, sunflower oil, fennel seeds and
lemon zest.

Add the dry mixture to the wet mixture, stirring until combined.

Pour the batter into the prepared tin, then stand the peach
halves up evenly along the centre of the cake.

Put the cake into the oven for 30–40 minutes, covering with foil
halfway through baking.

Leave to cool in the tin for 10 minutes, then turn onto a wire
rack and leave until cold. Peel off the paper.

Combine the icing ingredients in a bowl and pour over the cake.
Garnish with the sliced peach and lemon zest. Allow to set,
then serve.

150g ground almonds

50g buckwheat flour

1½ tsp baking powder

1 tsp bicarbonate of soda

¼ tsp Himalayan pink salt

2 eggs

1 tsp vanilla extract

80g (about 1 large) roughly
chopped peach

150ml agave syrup

60ml sunflower oil

2 tsp fennel seeds (optional)

zest of 1 lemon

2½ small peaches, sliced in
half and stoned

for the icing:

150g goats' milk or dairy-free
yoghurt

2 tbsp agave syrup

juice of ¼ lemon

1 tbsp coconut oil, melted

for the garnish:

1 peach, sliced

lemon zest

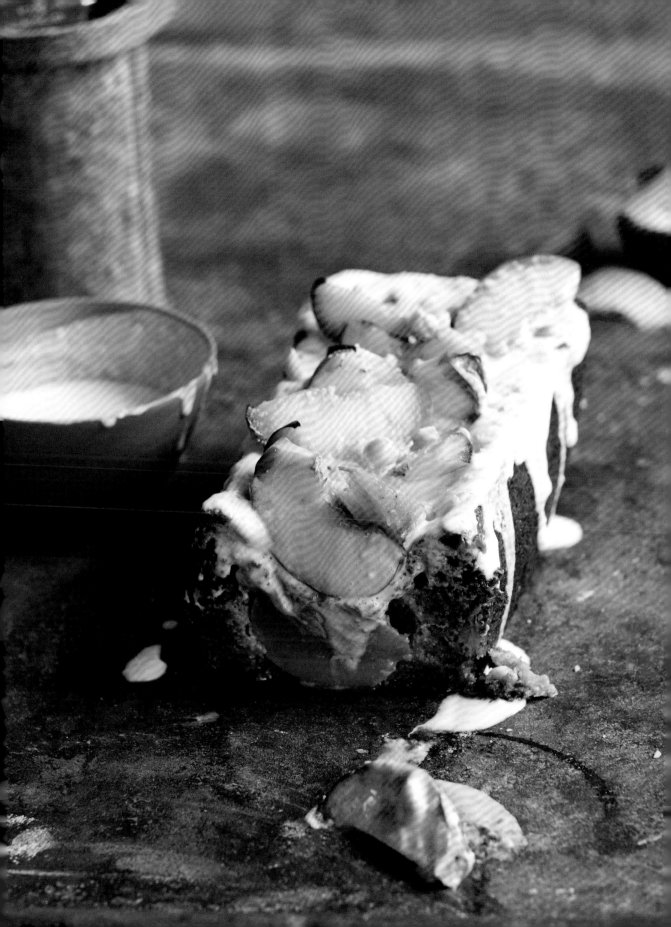

I grew up loving polenta cakes and I had a lot to
live up to writing this recipe. This cake is wonderfully moist
and so full of flavour. Put some candles on it and it's
also a great alternative birthday cake. I promise you will
love this one and it's simple to make.

SERVES 8–10

orange polenta cake

Preheat the oven to 180°C/160°C fan/gas mark 4 and line a 20cm cake tin with baking parchment.

In a bowl, combine the ground almonds, polenta, ground cinnamon, ground nutmeg, baking powder and salt.

In a separate bowl, cream together the vegan butter, coconut oil and palm sugar, then whisk in the eggs.

Tip the dry mixture into the wet, add the orange zest and combine.

Slice the skin and pith off the oranges and cut the flesh into 5mm slices. Line the bottom of the cake tin with the oranges so it is thoroughly covered. Pour the cake mixture over the top and smooth over with a spatula.

Bake in the oven for 35–40 minutes or until a skewer inserted into the middle of the cake comes out clean. Leave to cool before turning out of the tin onto a plate so that the oranges are on top.

While the cake is cooling, make the drizzle by combining all of the ingredients in a pan and simmering over a gentle heat for 5 minutes. Leave to cool for a minute or so before pouring or brushing it over the top of the cake.

Serve with a dollop of dairy-free cream or ice-cream (cashew cream would be delicious).

200g ground almonds
100g polenta
1 tsp ground cinnamon
½ tsp ground nutmeg
1 tsp baking powder
¼ tsp Himalayan pink salt
200ml coconut oil or 100ml coconut oil and 100g vegan butter
200g coconut palm sugar
4 eggs, beaten
zest of 2 oranges
3–4 oranges, depending on size

for the drizzle:
juice of 1 orange
1 tbsp date syrup
1 tbsp soft vegan butter

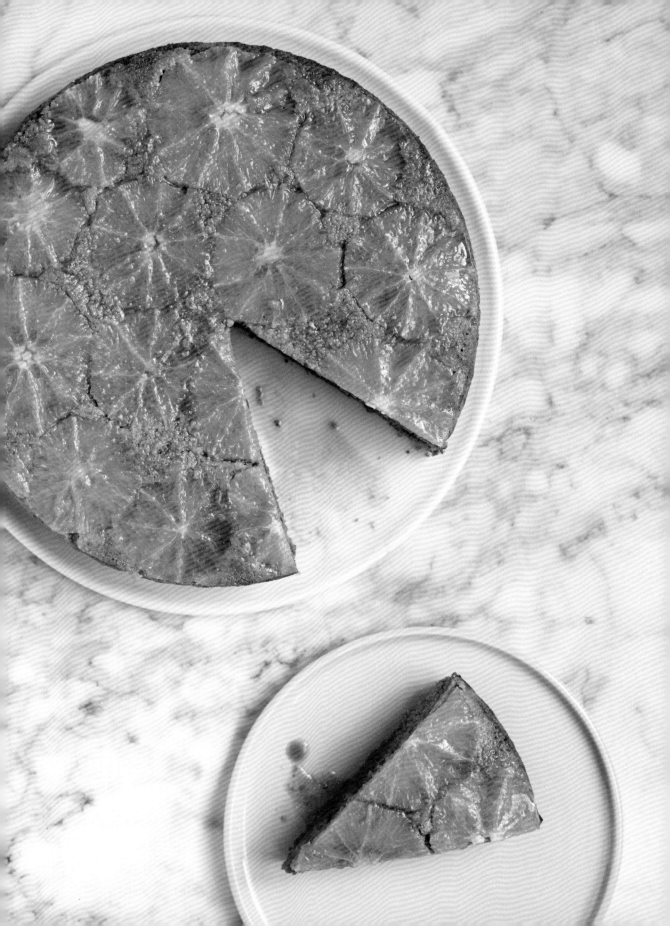

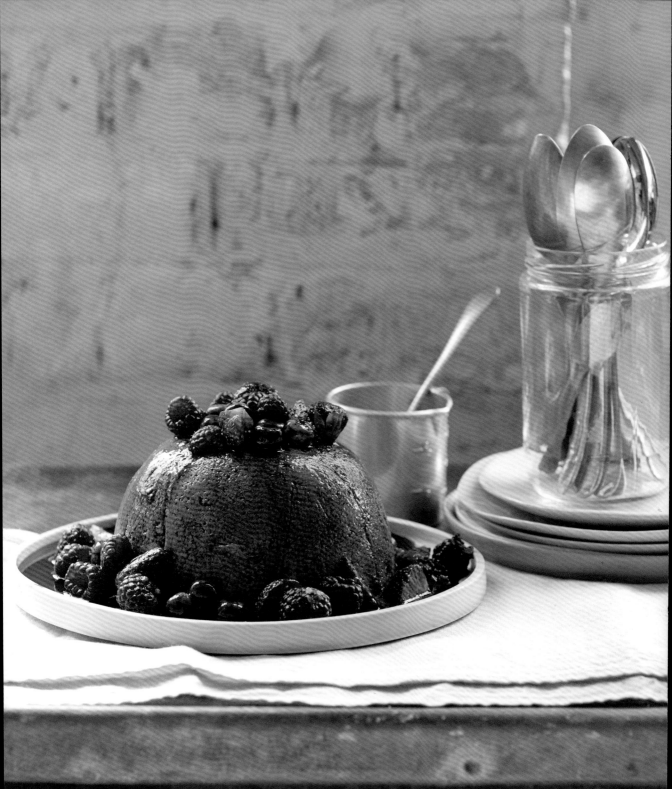

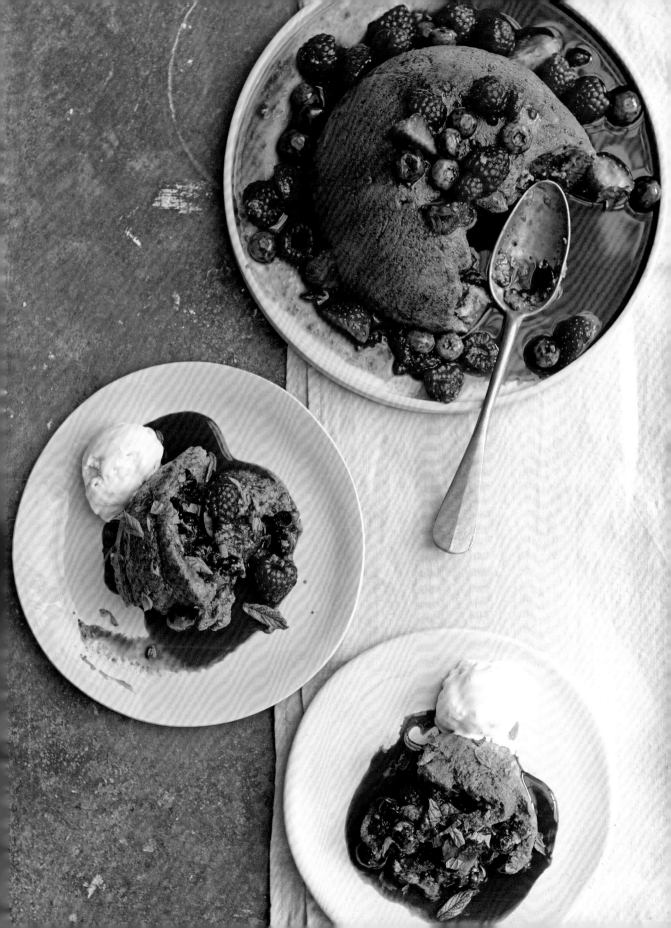

I know some might think that summer pudding is a little old school, but every time I go to my friends' house in the summer we have it – and I love, love, love it. It always looks so amazing, drizzled with that bright pink coulis and scattered with lots of extra berries. I therefore thought I ought to create a healthier version for those long summer days and dinners in the garden.

SERVES 6–8

summer pudding

Place the fruit, agave syrup and lime juice in a pan with 2 tablespoons water and simmer over a gentle heat for 4 minutes. The raspberries should have broken down and lots of delicious juice should be gathering at the bottom of the pan. Set a sieve over a bowl and drain the fruit.

Cut the crusts off the bread so that you have rectangles about 5cm wide and 10cm long. These will be used to line a 1 litre pudding bowl. Take one piece of bread at a time, dip it in the fruit juice and then place it up the side of the bowl. Repeat until you have gone all around the bowl, making sure that there are no gaps between each slice of bread. You might need to push the sides of each slice together a bit or cut some smaller fingers of bread to bridge any gaps. Finally, using a cutter, cut a circle of bread to fill the base of the bowl – use any offcuts to bridge further gaps as you don't want any of the fruit to escape.

Once the bowl is lined, pour the fruit and remaining juice into the centre of the bowl, then cover with more bread so as to seal the pudding.

The next step is to refrigerate the pudding overnight with a weight on top. I use a sideplate with an apple or two on top. The liquid should not overflow from the pudding, but put a plate under the bowl in the fridge just in case – you can always drizzle any overflow on top of the pudding when you serve.

Remove the pudding from the fridge when you are ready to serve and carefully flip it onto a plate. Drizzle any leftover juice on top and scatter the plate with some more berries and chopped mint.

Serve with a dollop of yoghurt.

250g raspberries
250g strawberries
120g blackcurrants
120g blueberries
3 tbsp agave syrup
zest and juice of ½ lime
6–8 slices gluten-free bread

Rhubarb will be really pink at the beginning of the season when it is nice and young – this is usually around February/March if you are in the UK. It will be slightly brown later in the year, but just as delicious. If you want to be sure of a really bright colour, just add a handful of blackcurrants, blueberries or blackberries to the compote.

SERVES 8–10

rhubarb tart

400g pink rhubarb, cut into 2cm by 5cm long strips
1 pear, peeled and cut into 2.5mm thick rounds
juice and zest of ½ lemon
4 tbsp agave syrup
4 star anise
3 tbsp toasted flaked almonds, to garnish

for the pastry:
250g ground almonds
1 egg, beaten
¼ tsp ground cinnamon

Preheat the oven to 200°C/180°C fan/gas mark 6 and line a 20cm tart tin with baking parchment.

First make the pastry. Put all of the ingredients for into a bowl with 1 tablespoon water and bring together with your hands to form a dough.

Place the dough in the centre of the prepared tin and press it out with your fingers until it neatly and evenly lines the bottom and sides. Bake in the oven for 10 minutes or until turning golden brown.

Meanwhile, put all of the rhubarb ingredients into a saucepan with 1½ tablespoons water and place over a medium heat. Put the lid on the pan and leave for 4 minutes before gently stirring – be as gentle as you can in order to retain the shape of the fruit. Put the lid back on the pan and cook for a further 2 minutes before removing from the heat. Gently stir again and, if soft and almost falling apart, the filling is ready. Rhubarb can be very tart at certain times of year, so add a little more sweetness if needed. Leave to cool.

Once the pastry case is cooked, pour in the filling and spread it out evenly.

Sprinkle the top with toasted almonds and serve with a dollop of dairy-free yoghurt, cream or ice-cream.

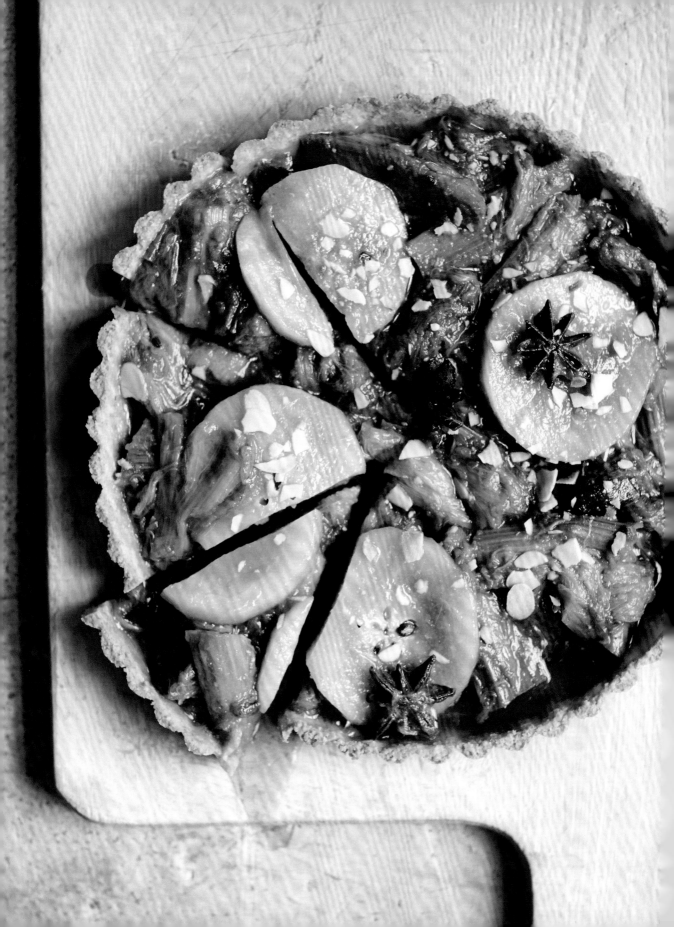

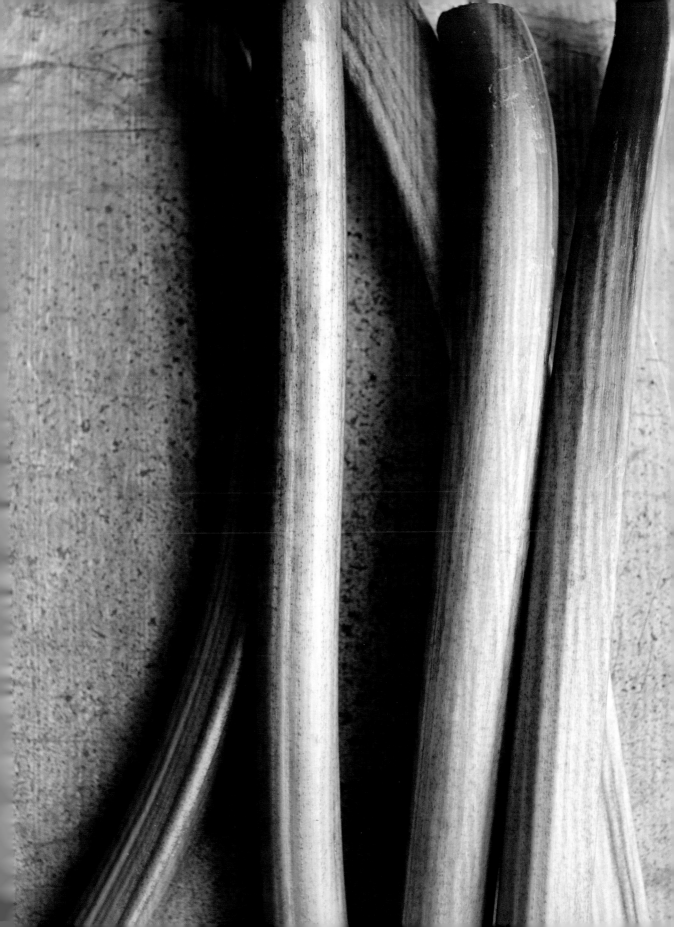

I have been wanting to write this recipe for a couple of years since I visited Vietnam. There I saw locals selling delicious-looking agar pots, so I have been plotting for a while now about how to develop them into little morsels of chocolaty deliciousness. These are great for a dinner party as you can quickly make them the night before and leave to set.

SERVES 2

white chocolate pots

Melt the cacao butter in a pan over a medium heat.

Put into a blender with the coconut cream, vanilla seeds or paste and the agave syrup and blend till velvety smooth.

Return the mixture to the pan and, before turning on the heat, sprinkle the agar over the top (do not stir). Bring to the boil, then stir in the agar. Simmer and stir for 10 minutes until all the agar is dissolved.

Pour into 2 ramekins or cups and put into the fridge to set for at least 3 hours. Garnish with the pomegranate seeds before serving.

50g raw cacao butter
160ml coconut cream (or the creamy top from a tin of coconut milk)
1 vanilla pod, seeds scraped out, or 1 tbsp vanilla paste
50ml agave syrup
1½ tsp agar flakes
pomegranate seeds, to garnish

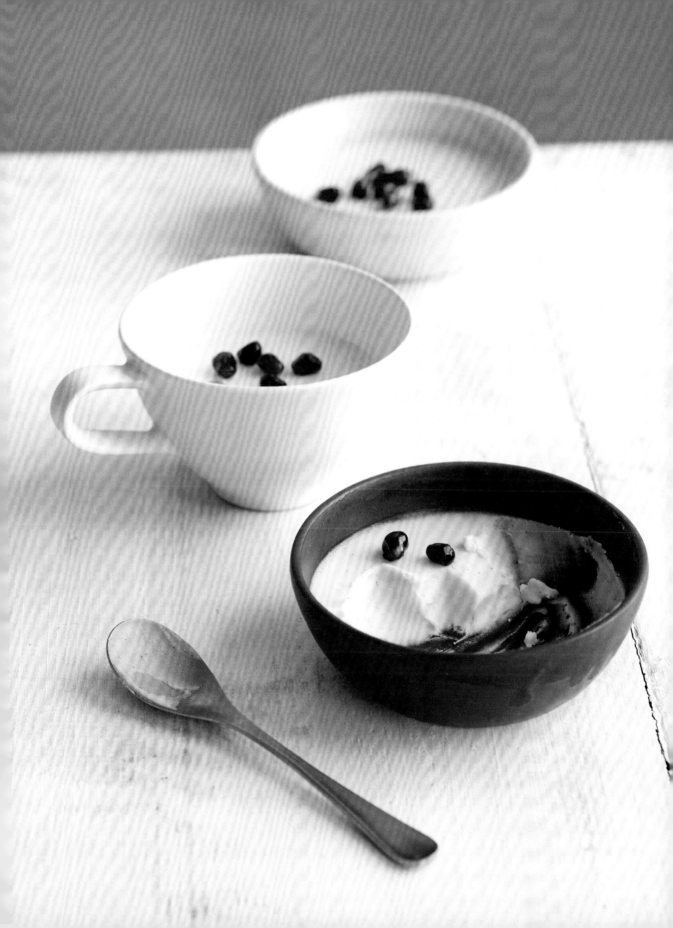

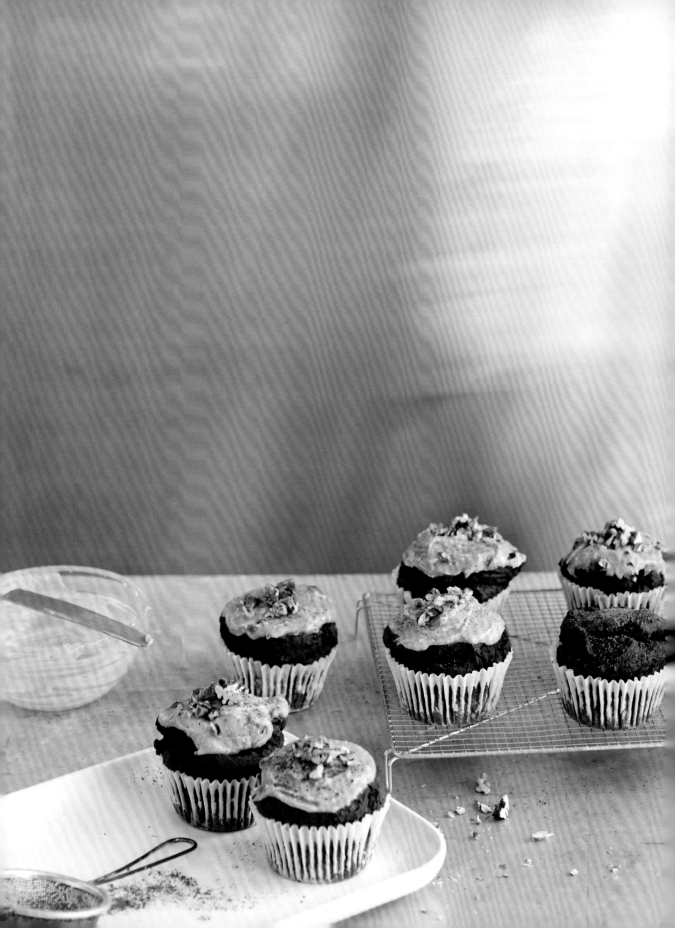

Muffins are a great treat and all the family loves them.
You can use sweet potato instead of parsnip for a sweeter texture
if you want to mix it up a bit. This is also a great one for hiding
extra veg in kids' meals! Oh, and the big kids love them too!

MAKES 9 MUFFINS

parsnip chocolate muffins

3 large parsnips or sweet potatoes, peeled and cut into 1cm chunks

260ml almond milk (bought or see page 52) or rice milk

100ml sunflower oil

100g teff flour

120g gluten-free plain flour

40g raw cacao powder

1½ tsp baking powder

1 tsp bicarbonate of soda

1 tsp xanthan gum

¼ tsp Himalayan pink salt

2 eggs

80g coconut palm sugar

60g date syrup, for extra sweetness (optional)

chopped walnuts, to garnish

for the cashew butter icing:

120g cashew butter

120ml agave syrup

Preheat the oven to 180°C/160°C fan/gas mark 4 and line a muffin tray with paper cases.

Steam the parsnip or sweet potato chunks until really soft. Transfer to a blender, add the almond milk and sunflower oil and whizz to a purée. Leave to cool down.

Put the flours and cacao powder into a bowl with the baking powder, bicarbonate of soda, xanthan gum and salt.

Beat the eggs and mix them into the parsnip mixture with the coconut palm sugar and date syrup (if using).

Add the dry mixture to the wet and stir well. Pour into the paper cases and bake for 20 minutes until a skewer inserted in the centre of a muffin comes out clean. Transfer to a rack to cool.

To make the icing, stir together the cashew butter and agave syrup with 4 teaspoons water. Spread over the top of the muffins when cool. Garnish with the chopped nuts.

The mixture for this dessert is dangerously good,
so wash the bowl as soon as possible to avoid excessive
licking! The pots are great for a dinner party as you
can make the mixture in advance and then just pop in
the oven while you are eating the main course.

SERVES 5

sticky toffee fondants

Preheat the oven to 180°C/160°C fan/gas mark 4 and grease 5 ramekins or pudding moulds with coconut oil.

Beat the eggs in a bowl and then whisk in the coconut oil, palm sugar and date syrup until really well combined with no lumps.

Put the dates into a bowl with the boiling water and leave to sit for 5 minutes to soften. Transfer to a blender with the vanilla extract and almond milk and blitz until smooth. Add to the egg mixture and whisk to combine.

Sift the flour, cacao powder and bicarbonate of soda into the mixture and fold through until totally incorporated.

Pour the batter equally into each ramekin. Place them in a baking tray and pour in enough boiling water to come halfway up the sides of the dishes. Bake in the oven for 19 minutes.

Make the sauce by melting the vegan butter with the coconut palm sugar over a low heat. Add the date syrup, stirring occasionally until combined and thick.

To serve, tip the risen puddings out on a plate and pour the sticky toffee sauce over the top. Serve with dairy-free vanilla ice-cream or yoghurt.

50g coconut oil, at room temperature, plus extra for greasing
2 eggs, beaten
70g coconut palm sugar
2 tbsp date syrup
100g dates, stoned
140ml boiling water
1 tsp vanilla extract
125ml almond milk (bought or see page 52)
120g gluten-free plain flour
1 tsp raw cacao powder
½ tsp bicarbonate of soda

for the sauce:
40g vegan butter
40g coconut palm sugar
80g date syrup

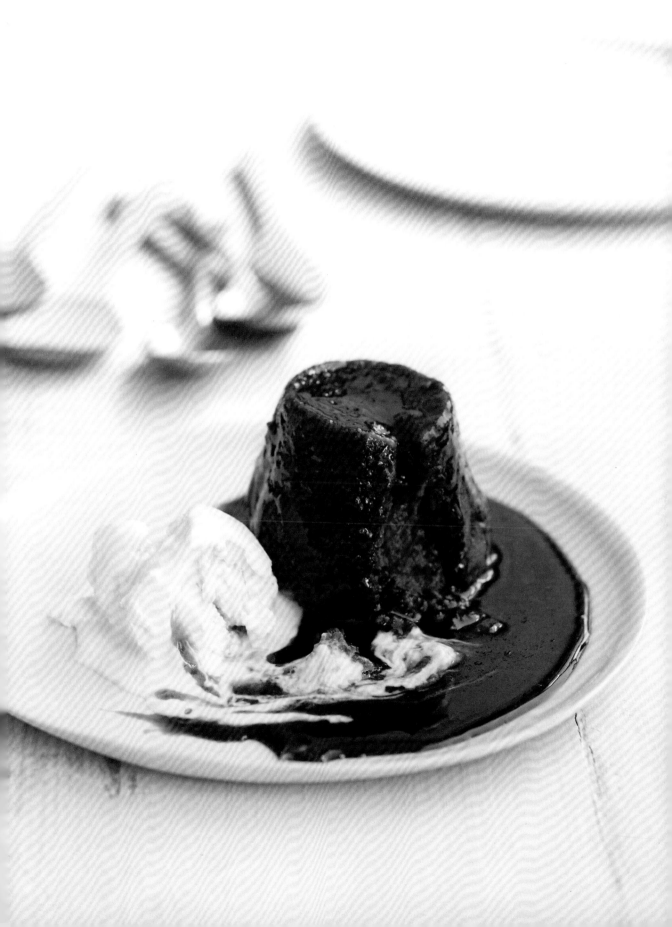

Everyone loves a good brownie and I have written quite a few recipes for them in my time, but these are based on a traditional recipe with a twist. In my first book *Honestly Healthy: Eat with Your Body in Mind, the Alkaline Way* I created a delicious sweet potato brownie: now let's see if the cauliflower addition will be the latest craze!

MAKES 9 BROWNIES

cauliflower protein brownies

Preheat the oven to 180°C/160°C fan/gas mark 4 and line a square 20cm brownie tin with baking parchment.

Steam the cauliflower florets over a medium heat until soft – this should take around 5–6 minutes. Once it has cooled a little, put the cauliflower into a blender. Melt the coconut oil or butter and add with the syrup, then blitz together to make a smooth purée. Set aside.

Sift all the dry ingredients into a bowl. In a separate bowl, whisk the egg and vanilla extract together.

Stir the cauliflower purée through the egg mixture and whisk until thoroughly combined. Gently fold the dry mixture into the wet, adding the chopped pecans at the end if you are opting to include them. Pour the mixture into your lined brownie tin.

To make the cashew swirl, stir together the cashew butter and agave syrup with 1 teaspoon water. Drizzle over the top of the brownie mixture and swirl using a teaspoon.

Bake in the oven for 20 minutes until a skewer inserted into a brownie comes out clean, though still a little moist.

You can make a double batch to go in the ice-cream on page 215.

180g cauliflower florets
80ml coconut oil or vegan butter
170g coconut blossom syrup
100g gluten-free plain flour
60g raw cacao powder
20g vegan protein powder
1 tsp bicarbonate of soda
¼ tsp Himalayan pink salt
1 egg
1 tbsp vanilla extract
60g pecans, roughly chopped (optional)

for the cashew butter swirl (optional):
30g cashew butter
30ml agave syrup

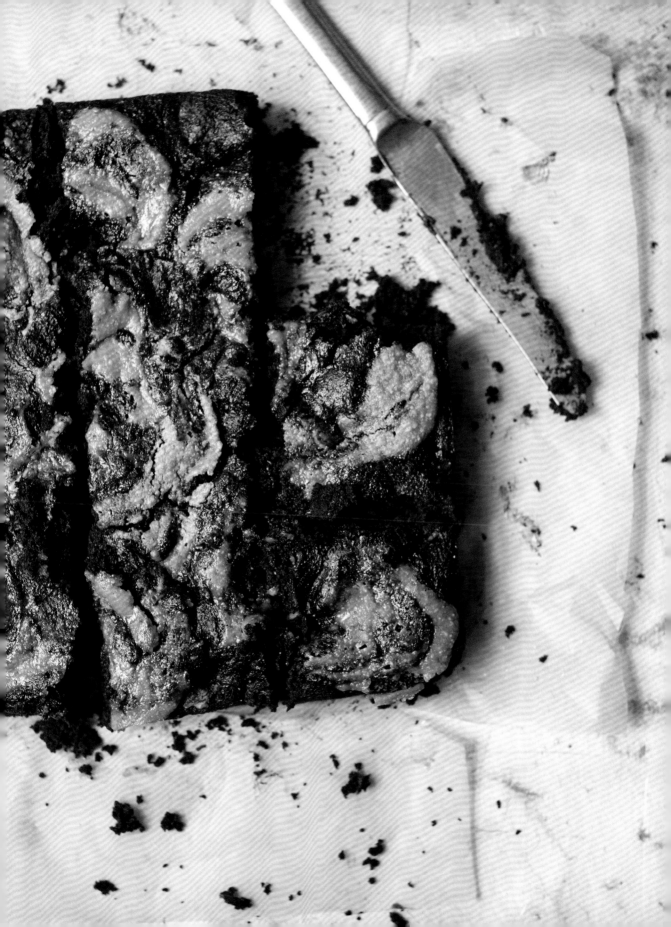

There's nothing more luxurious than breaking through the
chocolate shell of a truffle and sinking your teeth into
the creamy filling. The centres of these truffles have a slight
caramel taste and they are really simple to make.

MAKES 14 TRUFFLES

proper truffles

Soak the cashews in filtered water for at least 30 minutes until soft, then drain. If you don't have a strong blender, leave to soak for longer as this will help the truffles be silky smooth.

Put the cashews, coconut oil (it doesn't have to be melted), date syrup and cacao powder into a blender or a small food processor (a mini chopper would also work well). Start to blend and then add 2 tablespoons water, a tablespoon at a time. If using a blender, start on a low speed and leave for longer until you get a wonderful silky texture.

Line a baking sheet with baking parchment. Using 2 teaspoons or a melon-baller, scoop out balls of the mixture and place them on the lined sheet.

Put the truffles into the freezer for 15 minutes until solid enough for you to roll them into perfect balls in your palms. You can skip this step if you don't mind the truffles not being perfectly round. Or you can put the mixture into ice-cube moulds to make different shapes.

Make the chocolate shells by melting the cacao butter in a heatproof bowl set over, but not touching, a pan of simmering water. Take off the heat and either mix or blend in the syrup, vanilla and cacao powder until smooth. Dip the truffles into the sauce using a fork and replace them on the lined sheet. Once you have got to the end, the first ones will have set as they are so cold and you can re-dip them. There is even enough chocolate covering to triple-dip if you want. If not, use the remaining chocolate to put into ice-cube moulds to make little chocolates.

Sprinkle the truffles with cacao or matcha powder, or roll in chopped nuts after the second dipping.

Keep in the fridge until you're ready to serve them.

100g cashews

3 tbsp coconut oil

3 tbsp date syrup

1 tbsp raw cacao powder

for the chocolate shells:

80g raw cacao butter

1 tbsp date syrup

⅛ tsp vanilla extract

1 tbsp raw cacao powder, plus extra for rolling

matcha powder or finely chopped nuts, for rolling

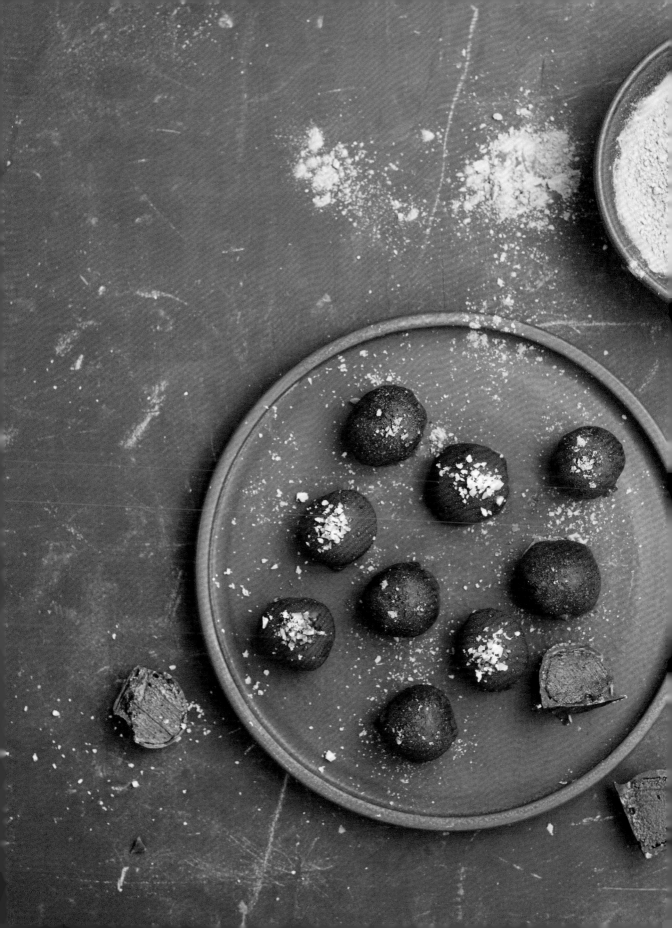

The most delicious smoothie and also perfect to make into little frozen bites for a sweet kids' treat. You can put the mixture into an ice-cream machine to make frozen yoghurt too.

SERVES 2 AS A SMOOTHIE OR MAKES 14 SMOOTHIE BITES

chamomile and raspberry smoothie bites

Start by brewing the chamomile tea bag in the water and allowing it to infuse for a good 5 minutes.

Next, put all of the remaining smoothie ingredients into a blender and blitz until smooth. Add the chamomile tea and serve as a smoothie at this point if you wish.

If you want to turn the smoothie into little bites that you can keep in your freezer, blend in the additional yoghurt, blueberries and lime zest and pour the mixture into an ice-cube tray. Store in the freezer and grab for a refreshing bite when you need one.

1 chamomile tea bag
60ml boiling water
100g frozen raspberries
70g banana
zest of ½ lime
1 tsp maca powder

for the smoothie bites:
60g yoghurt
20g blueberries
zest of ½ lime

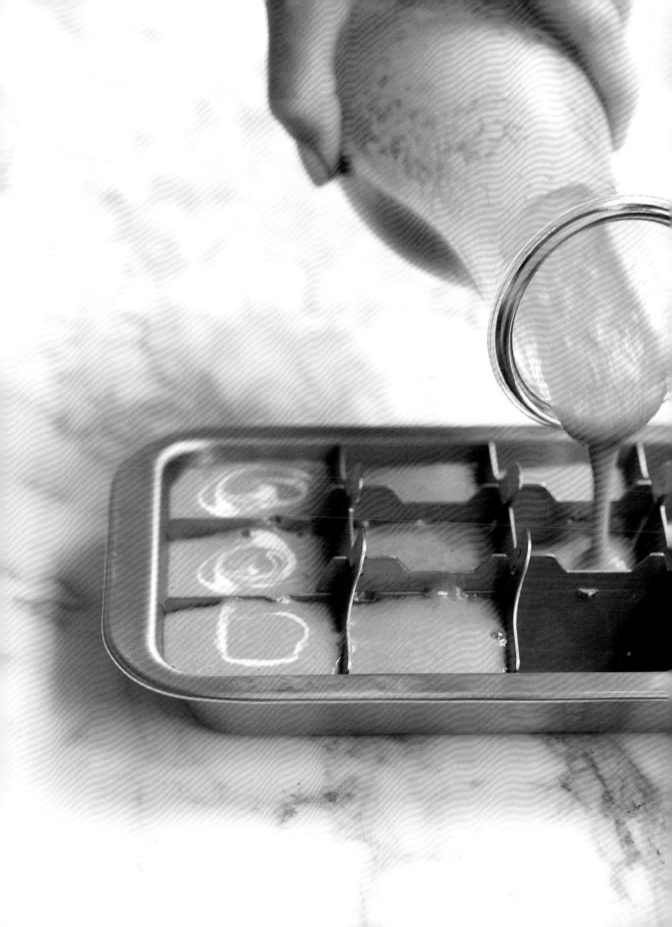

There's nothing I love more than watermelon. It's so refreshing, and the addition of rose water gives it a wonderful floral flavour. If you don't have rose water, you can leave it out or try using vanilla instead.

SERVES 8–10

watermelon rose sorbet

Make the watermelon juice by putting the flesh of the watermelon through a juicer.

Put the juice into a blender with the rose water and powdered agave and mix together for about a minute.

Pour into an ice-cream maker and churn according to the manufacturer's instructions. Alternatively, freeze in a shallow baking tray for 1 hour, then stir with a fork to break up the ice crystals. Repeat this step twice more, then freeze solid. Allow to soften slightly before serving.

1kg watermelon, juiced
   (850ml watermelon juice)
1 tsp rose water
3 tbsp agave powder or syrup
   of your choice

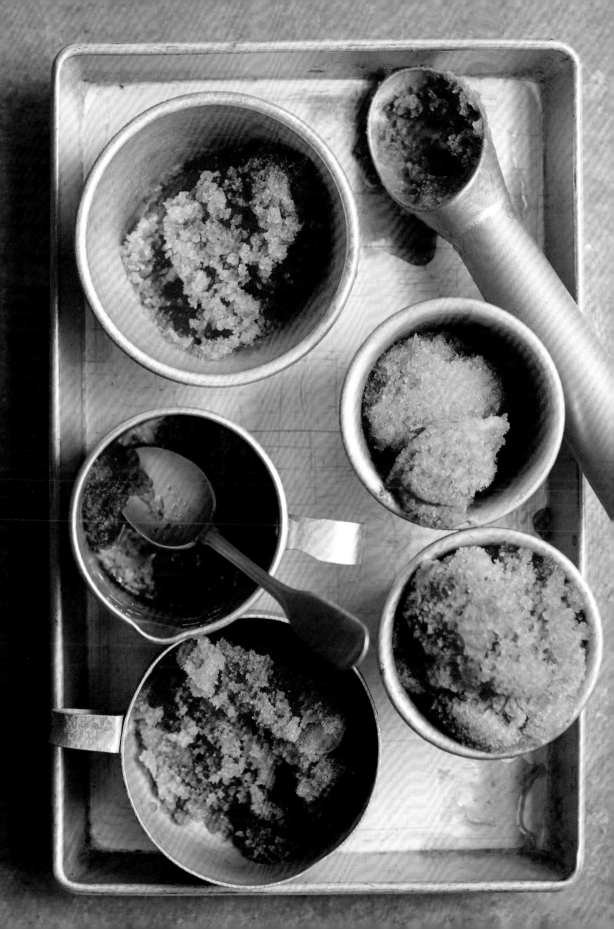

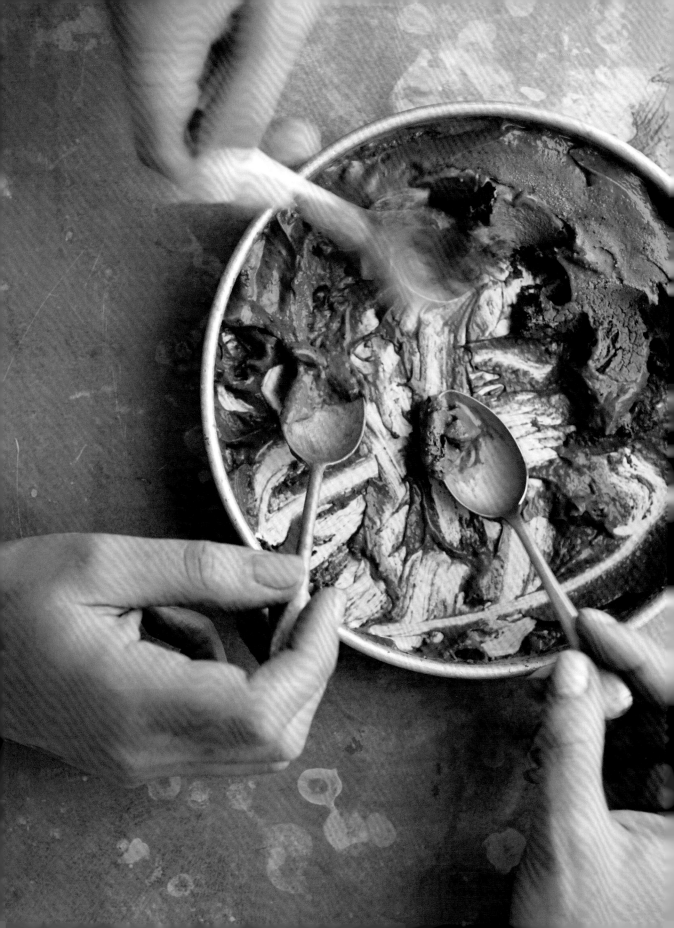

What can I say about this recipe other than if, like me, you love chocolate, you must try it! The brownies can be left out if you wish as the chocolate ice-cream part tastes wonderful just as it is.

SERVES 4–6 (MAKES 500ML)

double chocolate brownie ice-cream

400ml coconut milk

4 tbsp raw cacao powder

5 tbsp (85ml) date syrup

1 tsp xanthan gum

150g frozen Cauliflower protein brownies (see page 206)

If you are using an ice-cream maker, pre-cool the bowl.

Put the coconut milk, cacao powder and date syrup into a blender and blend until smooth. Add the xanthan gum and blend again to thicken it up and make it really creamy, though if the coconut milk is already really thick, don't add so much xanthan gum.

Get the brownies out of the freezer and chop them into 5mm square chunks (they must be frozen otherwise they will end up blending into the mixture).

Stir the brownies into the mixture, put into an ice-cream maker and freeze according to the manufacturer's instructions. Alternatively, freeze in a shallow baking tray for 1 hour, then stir with a fork to break up the ice crystals. Repeat this step twice more, then freeze solid. Allow to soften slightly before serving.

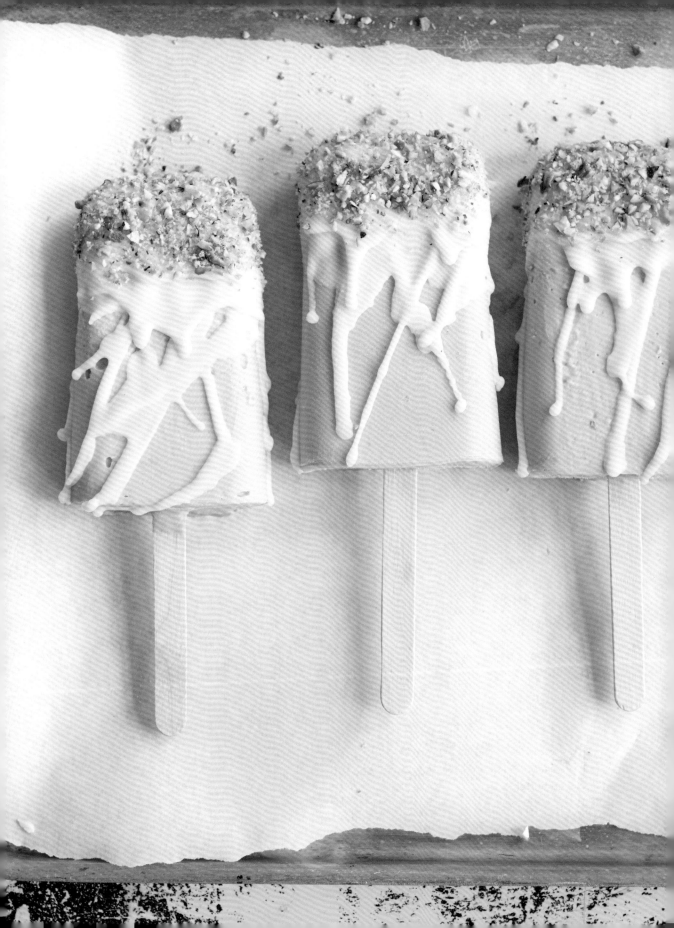

I used to love those Mini Milk ice lollies when I was younger
and thought it would be fun to create a healthier, dairy-free option
that the kids are going to love. This is probably one of the
quickest ice-creams you can make – it's just a case of blend and
freeze. I love that we can sneak some nutritious avocado in there
too. If you don't have ice-lolly moulds, just freeze the mixture
in a lidded plastic container and serve as ice-cream.

MAKES 4 POPS

avocado pops

2 ripe avocados, peeled and
   stones removed
juice of ½ lemon
60ml agave syrup
60g coconut oil, melted
¼ tsp vanilla extract
1 tbsp cashew butter or other
   nut butter
125ml almond milk
chopped pistachios, for
   dipping

*for the white chocolate
topping (optional):*
60g raw cacao butter
90g coconut cream (or the
   creamy top of a tin of
   coconut milk)
30g agave syrup

Put all of the ingredients (apart from the nuts) for the avocado
pops into a high-speed blender and blitz until velvety smooth.
Transfer to ice-lolly moulds and freeze for 2–3 hours until set.

If you want to add the white chocolate topping to the ice pops,
blitz all the ingredients for it in your blender. Spoon over the
lollies and dip them into the chopped nuts. Eat right away, or
return to the freezer to eat later.

One of the best ice-creams I have ever made! For a less expensive option you can use normal honey or agave or coconut blossom syrup instead of the manuka honey. I think manuka's health properties are fantastic, so I love the fact I can feel like I am being naughty, but I am boosting my immune system at the same time! I can shine my healthy halo.

SERVES 4

manuka pollen
maca ice-cream

Soak the almonds by covering them with enough water for them to float for a minimum of 30 minutes or, if you can, 2 hours, or, even better, overnight. Strain well.

Put the soaked almonds into a blender with 500ml water and blend until smooth.

Strain the mixture through a muslin bag over a large bowl. Keep the almond pulp to make the Almond pulp chewy bites on page 186.

Put the strained milk into a blender with the manuka honey, bee pollen, maca and vanilla. Blend until smooth.

Add the xanthan gum and blend for a few seconds. This will thicken the mixture and make it creamy.

Pour into an ice-cream maker and churn according to the manufacturer's instructions. Alternatively, freeze in a shallow baking tray for 1 hour, then stir with a fork to break up the ice crystals. Repeat this step twice more, then freeze solid. Allow to soften slightly before serving.

200g almonds
500ml water
105ml manuka honey
20g bee pollen
1 tsp maca powder
1 tsp vanilla extract
1 tsp xanthan gum

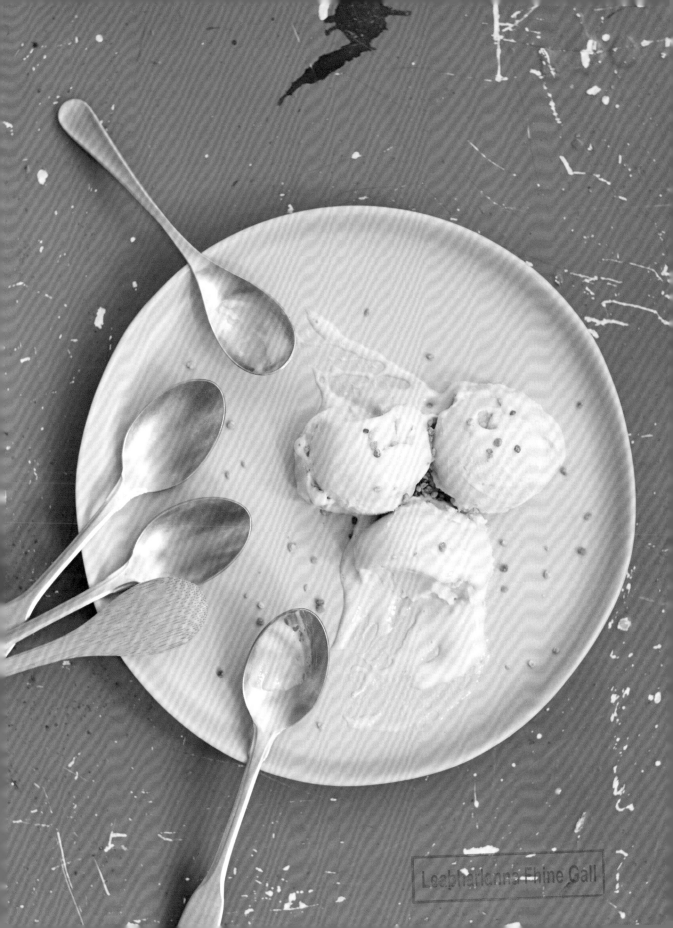

index

directory

Here are my favourite suppliers, most of which are in the UK.

Organic supermarkets & online suppliers

Infinity Foods www.infinityfoods.co.uk
Planet Organic www.planetorganic.com
Whole Foods www.wholefoodsmarket.com
Detox Your World www.detoxyourworld.com

Veg & fruit delivery services

Abel & Cole www.abelandcole.co.uk
Goodness Direct www.goodnessdirect.co.uk
Field to Fork Organics
www.fieldtoforkorganics.co.uk
Organic Delivery Company
www.organicdeliverycompany.co.uk
Riverford www.riverford.co.uk

Superfood suppliers

The Chia Co www.thechiaco.com.au
Evolution Organics www.evolutionorganics.co.uk
Natulya www.natulya.com
Organic Burst www.organicburst.com
The Synergy Company
www.thesynergycompany.com

Other products & suppliers

Alara (organic muesli) www.alara.co.uk
Biona (coconut oil) www.biona.co.uk
Bobs Red Mill www.bobsredmill.com
Clearspring (macrobiotic ingredients)
www.clearspring.co.uk
Coyo (coconut milk yoghurt) www.coyo.co.uk
Doves Farm (organic flour) www.dovesfarm.co.uk
Lucy Bee (extra virgin coconut oil)
www.lucybee.co.uk
OptiBac (probiotics) www.optibacprobiotics.co.uk
Nutribullet (smoothie-makers)
www.buynutribullet.co.uk
Rude Health (organic grains and drinks)
www.rudehealth.com
Tiana (virgin coconut oil) www.tiana-coconut.com
Vitamix (high-speed blenders) www.vitamix.co.uk

Fridge Fill

Honestly Healthy offers nationwide delivery of
ready-prepared alkaline Cleanse and Lifestyle
menus. www.honestlyhealthyfood.com

acknowledgements

I cannot thank you enough for buying this book. You help my dreams to come true for me to be able to follow my passion in life. Thank you to Nicky Ross and her wonderful team at Hodder for bringing this book to life.

To my unbelievable dream team Lisa, Lawrence, Cynthia, Dom, Rosannagh – I love having you involved in my books; they would not be the same without you.

A huge thank you to my Honestly Healthy team for holding the fort while I took so much time out to write and photograph the book, especially Simon!

To my husband who is always hungry, so learning to cook healthily in a hurry was a necessary part of being and staying married!

And finally to my wonderful friends who put up with being my taste testers ... it is sometimes a chore when the recipes are in their infant stages and they are not quite right yet. And a wonderful thank you to Magda and Jo for getting me picture perfect on my cover shoot.

Thank you x

First published in Great Britain in 2016 by Hodder & Stoughton
An Hachette UK company

1

Copyright © Natasha Corrett 2016
Photography copyright © Lisa Linder 2016

The right of Natasha Corrett to be identified as the Author of the Work has been asserted by her in accordance with the Copyright, Designs and Patents Act 1988.

A CIP catalogue record for this title is available from the British Library

Hardback ISBN 978 1 444 78181 6
Ebook ISBN 978 1 444 78182 3

Editorial Director: Nicky Ross
Editor: Sarah Hammond
Copy Editor: Kay Delves
Design & Art Direction: Lawrence Morton
Photographer: Lisa Linder
Food Styling: Natasha Corrett, Isla Mackenzie,
   Anna Burges-Lumsden, Clare Gray
Props Styling: Cynthia Inions
Layouts: Nicky Barneby

Printed and bound in China by C & C Offset Printing Co. Ltd.

Hodder & Stoughton policy is to use papers that are natural, renewable and recyclable products and made from wood grown in sustainable forests. The logging and manufacturing processes are expected to conform to the environmental regulations of the country of origin.

Hodder & Stoughton Ltd
Carmelite House
50 Victoria Embankment
London EC4Y 0DZ

www.hodder.co.uk